THE SELF-CONFIDENCE WORKBOOK

HELLO CONFIDENCE MY NAME IS

HELLO STRENGTH MY NAME IS

HELLO COURAGE MY NAME IS

HELLO FREEDOM MY NAME IS

HELLO CALM MY NAME IS

HELLO RESILIENCE MY NAME IS

HELLO OPENNESS MY NAME IS

HELLO GRATITUDE MY NAME IS

HELLO KINDNESS MY NAME IS

HELLO GENEROSITY MY NAME IS

HELLO CREATIVITY MY NAME IS

HELLO HAPPINESS MY NAME IS

HELLO COMPASSION MY NAME IS

THE
SELF-
CONFIDENCE
WORKBOOK

A Guide to Overcoming Self-Doubt and Improving Self-Esteem

Barbara Markway, PhD and Celia Ampel

FOREWORD BY TERESA FLYNN, PHD

ALTHEA
PRESS

For general information on our other products and services or to obtain technical support, please contact our Customer Care Department within the United States at (866) 744-2665, or outside the United States at (510) 253-0500.

Althea Press publishes its books in a variety of electronic and print formats. Some content that appears in print may not be available in electronic books, and vice versa.

Cover and Interior Designer: Merideth Harte
Editor: Susan Randol
Production Editor: Erum Khan
Illustrations: Merideth Harte

ISBN: Print 978-1-64152-148-2 | eBook 978-1-64152-149-9

QUICK START GUIDE

Is this book for you? Check the boxes that often describe you:

☐ Do you keep your thoughts to yourself, assuming you don't have anything important to share?

☐ If you're not completely sure you can do something, do you think, "Why bother trying?"

☐ Do you avoid talking to people, worrying that you'll have nothing to say or come across as awkward?

☐ Do you second-guess yourself frequently?

☐ Do you apologize excessively, even when you haven't done anything wrong?

☐ Do you hold yourself back from taking risks because you're afraid you'll fail?

☐ When you feel you didn't perform well, do you spend lots of time afterward ruminating on your mistakes?

☐ Do you give up easily?

☐ Does your inner voice tell you, "I'm not good enough; I can't do it"?

☐ Do you avoid pursuing some of your goals and dreams because of fear and self-doubt?

If you checked several of the boxes, read on to learn about proven strategies to build your self-confidence.

HELLO MY NAME IS CONFIDENCE

HELLO MY NAME IS STRENGTH

HELLO MY NAME IS COURAGE

HELLO MY NAME IS CALM

HELLO MY NAME IS FREEDOM

HELLO MY NAME IS RESILIENCE

HELLO MY NAME IS OPENNESS

HELLO MY NAME IS GRATITUDE

HELLO MY NAME IS KINDNESS

HELLO MY NAME IS CREATIVITY

HELLO MY NAME IS GENEROSITY

HELLO MY NAME IS HAPPINESS

HELLO MY NAME IS COMPASSION

To you, the reader:

May you have the confidence to
show up, stand up, and speak up.

The world needs your gifts.

HELLO MY NAME IS CONFIDENCE

HELLO MY NAME IS STRENGTH

HELLO MY NAME IS COURAGE

HELLO MY NAME IS FREEDOM

HELLO MY NAME IS CALM

HELLO MY NAME IS RESILIENCE

HELLO MY NAME IS OPENNESS

HELLO MY NAME IS GRATITUDE

HELLO MY NAME IS KINDNESS

HELLO MY NAME IS GENEROSITY

HELLO MY NAME IS CREATIVITY

HELLO MY NAME IS HAPPINESS

HELLO MY NAME IS COMPASSION

CONTENTS

FOREWORD

RESEARCH HAS SHOWN that self-confidence is linked to almost everything we want in life: success at work, secure relationships, a positive sense of self, and happiness. But what is self-confidence? Why does it appear to be so mysterious? Why does it seem like other people have it and we don't?

In my work as a psychologist, I often find low self-confidence is a common denominator regardless of the problem people come in for. For example, I worked with a young man who suffered from loneliness but was afraid to ask anyone out on a date. He didn't believe he was attractive enough, or interesting enough, or fun enough. Another client I worked with was a successful business-woman who was experiencing severe burnout. She took on too many projects, didn't delegate well, and was prone to perfectionism. Underneath it all, she felt like an impostor, and she overworked herself to compensate. Both, at their core, lacked self-confidence.

My clients typically say, "I don't feel confident, so I couldn't possibly . . . [insert desired goal here]." Can you relate? Not many of us are taught how confidence truly works. We get it backwards: We believe we have to wait until we feel confident before we can act confidently. That is why I am so excited you have this book in your hands. You are finally going to learn the truth about confidence: what it is, where it comes from, and how to master the rules of the confidence game. No matter your personality or circumstances, this workbook will show you how to move from passivity to actively pursuing your goals.

As a therapist, I'm also excited to have this book as a resource. I frequently assign reading and outside activities to my clients, and *The Self-Confidence Workbook* fills a much-needed gap. It's grounded in the latest advances in

Cognitive Behavioral Therapy (CBT) and Acceptance and Commitment Therapy (ACT), yet it's reader-friendly, presenting the skills you need in easy-to-digest nuggets. Each chapter contains valuable exercises and includes highly practical action items. Although the book is grounded in science, you won't get bogged down in technical jargon or long explanations of theory.

I first met Dr. Barbara Markway when we both worked at the Anxiety Disorders Center at the St. Louis University School of Medicine over twenty years ago. I was a psychologist and she was a postdoctoral fellow completing advanced training in Cognitive Behavioral Therapy. A skilled and caring therapist, she was also passionate about writing. She was adept at taking scientific information and putting it in everyday language in order to help people beyond her own office.

During her time at the Center for OCD and Anxiety-Related Disorders, we co-authored, along with Dr. Alec Pollard and Dr. Cheryl Carmin, *Dying of Embarrassment: Help for Social Anxiety and Phobia*. Dr. Markway went on to write two other books for those suffering with shyness and social anxiety, *Painfully Shy* and *Nurturing the Shy Child*. In addition to her writing, she maintained a clinical practice in a number of settings, from outpatient mental health clinics to private practice.

Dr. Markway has helped thousands of people build confidence and accomplish things they never dreamed possible, and I can't think of a better guide for you in your own journey to self-confidence.

I wish you well on this journey.

Teresa Flynn, PhD
Psychologist and Author
Adjunct Professor of Psychology
Washington University, St. Louis, Missouri

INTRODUCTION

I HAVE A CONFESSION TO MAKE. If you asked me to describe myself, I'd use words such as *creative*, *kind*, *persistent*, and *hardworking*. But I don't think *self-confident* would even make the top 10 list of adjectives. That's because when I've historically thought of self-confidence, I've pictured someone flashy and bold, and I'm definitely not that. But what I've learned is that self-confidence doesn't have to look flashy. In fact, self-confidence has more to do with inner resolve than with outward bravado.

I actually have a healthy degree of self-confidence now, but it wasn't always that way. I grew up a shy, anxious kid who rarely spoke to people other than my close friends and family. Although bright, I never raised my hand in class to answer a question. I was too afraid even to ask to go to the bathroom. In high school, my math teacher announced to the whole class that I was the quietest kid he had ever taught in his entire teaching career. I was humiliated. Everyone turned around to look at me, and I could feel my face turning hot and red. I went on to college and continued to do well in school, but never dated or enjoyed much of a social life. I was always interested in psychology, partly because I was trying to understand myself. Why was I so shy and quiet? Why couldn't I just break out of my shell? Why couldn't I just be myself? I ended up in graduate school studying clinical psychology and earned my PhD.

Along the way, I went through a lot of psychotherapy that proved very helpful. I learned to speak up. I learned my opinion mattered. I also learned it was okay to be wrong. I even mustered up the courage to ask my now-husband of nearly 30 years out on a date. Somewhere along the way, I became self-confident—I just didn't label it as such.

I became a psychotherapist and was naturally drawn to helping people with anxiety. There is nothing more satisfying than helping people learn to believe in themselves and master something that once terrified them. I also went on to write three books on overcoming social anxiety and shyness.

Over my nearly 30-year career, whether it's been through face-to-face therapy sessions or through my writing, I have helped thousands of people learn to be more self-confident. They've all had something they wanted to do—something important, something they valued—but they were letting fear, doubt, and lack of confidence stand in their way. I'm guessing that if you've picked up this book, you may be in the same boat.

The good news is you're completely normal. I know when you're in the middle of a self-confidence crisis, it can seem like you're the only one struggling and that everyone else has it all together. But you're not alone, and this book will help. I'm excited to share with you all I've learned about building a meaningful, confident life.

I've enlisted the help of a friend and fellow writer, Celia Ampel. As a shy person, she started reading my work while studying journalism at the University of Missouri. As a reporter, she has also overcome many of the fears that used to overwhelm her as a kid—she no longer has to write out a script before making a phone call—and much of that progress is thanks to the tools you'll learn in this book. Although we're creating this book as a team, we know it can be confusing to switch back and forth between us, alerting the reader to who is saying what. So this book is written in my "voice."

While I hope this book will be helpful, I'm not suggesting that after reading it you will never doubt yourself again. It's not realistic to expect yourself to have unshakable self-confidence. Everyone struggles with self-doubt and lack of confidence from time to time. It's part of being human. What this book *will* do is teach you tools, grounded in science, to help keep your self-critic from jerking you around. You'll learn to set meaningful goals, deal with your inner doubts, and not second-guess yourself all the time. You'll be able to walk out on that stage, ask for a raise, write that blog post, or ask someone out on a date. I'm not saying it will always be easy, but it will be possible. And you won't be on the journey alone. I'll be guiding you all the way.

HELLO CONFIDENCE MY NAME IS

HELLO STRENGTH MY NAME IS

HELLO COURAGE MY NAME IS

HELLO FREEDOM MY NAME IS

HELLO CALM MY NAME IS

HELLO RESILIENCE MY NAME IS

HELLO OPENNESS MY NAME IS

HELLO GRATITUDE MY NAME IS

HELLO KINDNESS MY NAME IS

HELLO GENEROSITY MY NAME IS

HELLO CREATIVITY MY NAME IS

HELLO HAPPINESS MY NAME IS

HELLO COMPASSION MY NAME IS

PART 1

SETTING THE STAGE

Tackling the demons of self-doubt is a brave and worthy pursuit. At times, you're going to feel discouraged or scared, but that just means you're really trying, which is infinitely better than allowing low self-confidence to keep you on the sidelines of life. The first two chapters of this book will lay the foundation for the work you'll do to bolster your self-confidence in later sections.

In chapter 1, we'll dismantle common misconceptions about self-confidence and learn what it really is, where it comes from, and most importantly, that you are totally capable of attaining it. You'll get a sense of how confident you are right now, setting a baseline from which to measure your growth. You'll see how different life can be when you have the gusto to go for your goals.

In chapter 2, you'll examine what's really important to you, identifying the values closest to your heart so that you can make an action plan that aligns with who you want to be. Then you'll set goals, envisioning a life where self-doubt doesn't hold you back from advancing in your career, setting a good example for your kids, facing conflict, building strong relationships, or making a difference in your community. You'll learn about the science behind the tried-and-true methods this book is based on, all of which will help you get out of your own way and be the best version of yourself. So give yourself a pat on the back for getting started, and let's go!

CHAPTER 1

UNDERSTANDING SELF-CONFIDENCE

. . . .

"IF YOU HEAR A VOICE WITHIN YOU SAYING, 'YOU CANNOT PAINT,' THEN BY ALL MEANS PAINT AND THAT VOICE WILL BE SILENCED."

—VINCENT VAN GOGH

If you had all the confidence in the world, what would you do?

> Larry would start that novel he's been wanting to write.
> Rita would talk to her boss about the promotion she was
> promised six months ago.
> LaShonda would talk to her partner about how she's
> been feeling disconnected in the relationship.

What about you?

What would you do if you had all the confidence in the world? Take a minute and jot down the first thing that comes to mind.

Larry, Rita, and LaShonda don't want confidence simply for the sake of confidence.

Larry wants to express his creativity.
Rita wants to stick up for herself.
LaShonda wants to improve her relationship.

My guess is there's something you want, but self-doubt and insecurity are holding you back. That's why I wrote this workbook: to help you take steps toward being your best self.

In this chapter, I will define self-confidence and what it can do for you. Together, we'll explore some myths about what confidence looks like and explain its true origins. Then we'll examine where low self-confidence comes from: Which life experiences might have shaped your beliefs about yourself? At the end of the chapter, you'll take a self-assessment to determine your current level of confidence.

Start at the Source

Confidence is a mysterious quality. It's one of those things we'd all like to have, but what does it really mean to be confident?

Most of the time, it's defined as a feeling: "I feel confident I can run the 5K in 28 minutes." We typically associate this type of confidence with calm, ease, and assurance. When we feel confident, we anticipate being successful.

The problem with defining confidence as a feeling is that in practice it becomes a catch-22: If you don't feel confident, you're not likely to try.

There's another definition of confidence, although it's not as common. The Latin roots of confidence mean "with trust." Acting with trust usually means you're not completely certain of what you're doing—you're taking a leap of faith. In other words, it's what we do that matters, not so much how we feel when we're doing it.

We can see this principle in action by considering the example of Darnell, a man who ordinarily kept to himself. Darnell was passionate about a zoning issue affecting his neighborhood, but he didn't like attention and feared standing up in front of the city council to speak his mind.

However, after reminding himself of how important the issue was to him and his neighbors, Darnell showed up to the meeting and said his piece, even as his hands shook. He didn't wait for his nervousness to subside entirely—then he might never have been able to speak. Instead, he gathered courage by rooting himself in his beliefs and then taking action.

In this book, I'll use the following definition of self-confidence: *the willingness to take steps toward valued goals, even if you're anxious and the outcome is unknown.* True self-confidence is part courage, part competence, with a healthy dose of self-compassion mixed in. I'll break this definition into bite-size chunks as we move through the workbook. For now, the key points to remember are:

Actions come before feelings.
Actions are guided by values—the things you care about.
Process is more important than outcome.

WHERE CONFIDENCE COMES FROM

Our beliefs about ourselves are often shaped by those around us, including family, friends, and media messages, sociologists have found. But that doesn't mean your level of confidence is out of your control—in fact, it's quite the contrary.

Confidence comes from being grounded in your sense of self: remembering who you are, what you value, and the hard work you've put in.

Studies show that a simple thought exercise can help people decrease their anxiety ahead of having to perform a task in a high-stakes situation. In research led by psychologists David Creswell and David Sherman, participants were asked to take a moment to reflect on a core value—say, being a good friend or respecting the environment. Then, each person wrote about a memory of a time they embodied that value.

Those who did the exercise had far lower adrenaline levels heading into stressful situations, such as exams or public speeches, than those who didn't—even if the core values weren't at all relevant to the task at hand. What mattered was that the participants were contemplating a deep truth about themselves, rather than a hollow slogan, such as "I'm the best." I'll walk you through some similar exercises in chapter 2.

A connection to our authentic selves can also help us take some of the pressure off ourselves going into scary situations. When Tanya was set to give a toast at her sister's wedding, she was extraordinarily anxious about having all eyes on her. She worried about her hands shaking and her voice quavering. But when she thought about it, impressing all 200 guests with a perfectly delivered speech didn't truly matter to her. What was really important to Tanya was showing her sister and new brother-in-law how much she loved them and hoped for their happiness. With that principle in mind, she stood up at the ceremony with mostly calm nerves and gave a heartfelt toast that strengthened the bonds she valued the most.

Of course, not all self-doubt is a bad thing! Sometimes fear is a signal that we haven't prepared enough for the big presentation, the recital, or the interview. Practicing what you plan to say and do will give your mind something to fall back on when the pressure is high. The voice of self-doubt may also be saying we need to get more information, move in a different direction, or take a break.

But we often err on the side of hesitating too much. Once you've put in the hours of practice, you should be able to take action without obsessing over what might go wrong. In this book, we will provide you with the tools to adjust your mind-set to a place of confidence.

WHAT IT MEANS TO BE CONFIDENT

When you envision a confident person, you might think of someone who takes big, bold actions, like running for office or proposing marriage on the jumbotron. But there can be a lot of boldness and bravery in small steps.

QUIET CONFIDENCE

"There's zero correlation between being the best talker and having the best ideas."

—SUSAN CAIN

Have you ever felt like you had a great idea, but you weren't confident enough to share it? Maybe you thought you weren't outgoing enough, assuming that only talkative people get noticed.

It's true that society tends to place more value on extroversion. That means if you're an introvert, you may have struggled more with self-confidence, feeling like you don't fit in or are somehow defective.

Fortunately, thanks in part to Susan Cain's best-selling book, *Quiet: The Power of Introverts in a World That Can't Stop Talking*, introverts are coming into their own, and many of the myths about introversion are being challenged.

So, if you're a self-described introvert, don't worry. You are not going to have to change your personality to enjoy greater self-confidence. As Mahatma Gandhi wisely said, "In a gentle way, you can shake the world."

Confidence isn't something you have to possess every moment of every day. Nor should you expect to jump instantly into perfect self-assurance tomorrow. Instead, confidence is a choice to take steps to act in line with your values.

Those incremental changes build on themselves, both through our own feelings of accomplishment and reinforcement from others. But in order to set off that virtuous cycle, it's important to practice self-compassion: speaking to yourself with the kindness and patience you would show a loved one or a child.

For example, when Sofia moved to a new city with her husband, she knew she wanted to make more friends. She heard about a free poetry workshop at a local café, and although she enjoyed writing, she was hesitant to attend. What if she had to read her amateur poetry in front of everyone?

Sofia told herself it was okay just to go, even if she didn't speak up as much as other people. She introduced herself to a few others at the table and participated in the writing prompts, but stayed silent when the instructor asked for volunteers to read their poems. At the very end of the event, she raised her hand once to thank the teacher for the workshop.

On the way home, Sofia had a choice. She could let her inner critic run wild, saying, *You're such a weirdo . . . You sat there silently the whole night . . . People probably wondered why you were even there, and they found you unfriendly, too!* Those thoughts would probably convince her the night had been a failure and that she should never go back to the monthly meetings.

Or, instead, Sofia could congratulate herself. She could see attending the workshop as a big, bold step—hey, by thanking the instructor, she even spoke in front of the whole group! Next month, she can set a goal to go back, have more conversations with the other participants, and maybe even share her writing. Her self-compassion, a concept we'll explore more later in the book, will allow her confidence to grow.

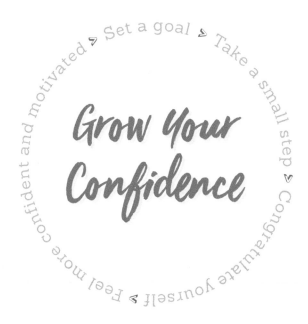

As Sofia shows us, you don't have to change your personality to be confident. There is emotional complexity in confidence. You can be strong and bold, but also honest, kind, and comfortable.

Think about a time you let your inner critic stop you from trying something new. What could you say to yourself next time to be more self-compassionate?

WHAT CONFIDENCE IS NOT

Some of us fear confidence because we don't want to start stepping on other people's toes, taking up too much space, or just plain being a jerk. But confidence isn't the same as arrogance or narcissism. In fact, when we feel confident in ourselves, we often become *less* self-absorbed. When we stop worrying so much about how we're coming across, we can pay more attention to those around us.

Confidence is not about being the one who speaks the loudest or who dominates every moment. It's also not about having a fancy car or other symbols of wealth or status. It's about being rooted in who you really are, freeing up your mind from obsessive worry and self-doubt.

Confidence is about being rooted in who you really are.

Staying grounded in a sense of self includes having a realistic view of your strengths as well as your weaknesses. Confidence can be a helpful buffer against internalizing unhelpful criticism that doesn't have much to do with what you really value—for instance, you can let your mother-in-law's comment about your hairstyle roll off your back. That doesn't mean you ignore all criticism because you believe you're already perfect.

THE CONFIDENCE CURVE

Did you ever think you could have too much self-confidence? Let's look at an example that shows how self-confidence is all about balance. Too little confidence and you avoid trying new things, pass on taking even small risks, and miss out on engaging in activities that would make life more meaningful and enjoyable. Too much confidence—confidence not grounded in reality—can get you into trouble.

Let's look at this in action. Imagine you're scheduled to give a presentation. The chart below shows the difference between being confident and overconfident.

Confident	Overconfident
I am well prepared. I know I can do this.	I know this material so well, I'm not going to prepare.
I will do my best to connect with the audience.	The audience better love me.
I might not give a flawless presentation, but I'll learn from my mistakes.	I'm too perfect to make a mistake.
I'll listen to the audience's questions and then thoughtfully respond.	I'll just wing the Q and A part.
It's OK if I don't have all the answers.	I'm the expert. I know everything.

Although this example might seem extreme, it illustrates some important points. First, confidence involves preparation. You have to put in the needed work ahead of time. Second, confidence doesn't mean you won't make mistakes; you will, but the mistakes won't crush you. You'll take the feedback and learn from it. And finally, confidence involves listening.

On the contrary, a confident person can accept helpful feedback and act on it without getting defensive. When your sense of self-worth is no longer on the table, you can handle criticism or even outright rejection without allowing it to break you.

By the same token, confidence doesn't mean you mow other people down when a conflict arises. It's possible to speak your mind with conviction and still make room to listen to someone else's point of view, and even reach a compromise.

Lastly, confidence doesn't mean you won't fail. It doesn't mean you're always smiling or that you never experience anxiety or self-doubt. Instead, it means you know you can handle those feelings and push through them to conquer the next challenge.

Who is someone you think embodies confidence and why?

_____

_____

_____

_____

Reasons for Low Self-Confidence

The most important thing to know about low self-confidence is that it is not your fault. Many people struggle with negative self-perception for a variety of reasons. This book applies to people with a wide range of self-confidence issues and differing levels of severity. If you have been diagnosed with an anxiety disorder or depression, you can use this book in conjunction with your other therapies.

The factors that contribute to low self-confidence combine and interact differently for each person. Your genes, cultural background, childhood experiences, and other life circumstances all play a role. But don't lose heart—although we can't change the experiences in our past that shaped us, there is plenty we can do to alter our thoughts and expectations to gain more confidence.

GENES AND TEMPERAMENT

Some of what molds our self-confidence is built into our brains at birth. I mention these factors not to overwhelm you but to let you know that you shouldn't blame yourself for your self-image.

Studies have shown that our genetic makeup affects the amount of certain confidence-boosting chemicals our brain can access. Serotonin, a neurotransmitter associated with happiness, and oxytocin, the "cuddle hormone," can both be inhibited by certain genetic variations. Somewhere between 25 and 50 percent of the personality traits linked to confidence may be inherited.

Some aspects of our behavior also stem from our temperament. If you're naturally more hesitant and watchful, especially in unfamiliar circumstances, you may have a tendency called *behavioral inhibition*. When you're confronted with a situation, you stop and check to see if everything seems the way you expected it to be. If something appears awry, you're likely to move away from the situation.

Behavioral inhibition is not all bad. We need some people in the world who don't impulsively jump into every situation. If you're a cautious and reserved person, self-confidence may have eluded you. But once you understand yourself and the tools in this book, you'll be able to work with your temperament and not fight it.

LIFE EXPERIENCES

A number of individual experiences can lead to feeling completely unsure of yourself or even worthless. Here, I'll discuss a few.

Trauma. Physical, sexual, and emotional abuse can all significantly affect our feelings of self-worth. If you find yourself replaying memories of abuse or otherwise feeling tormented by or ashamed of your experiences, please consider seeking treatment from a licensed clinician.

Parenting style. The way we were treated in our family of origin can affect us long after childhood. For instance, if you had a parent who constantly belittled you, compared you to others, or told you that you would never amount to anything, you likely carry those messages with you today. A parent's struggles with mental health and substance abuse can also change your relationship with the world.

Bullying, harassment, and humiliation. Childhood bullying can leave a mark on your confidence when it comes to looks, intellectual and athletic abilities, and other areas of your life. Humiliating experiences in adulthood, including workplace harassment or a peer group that disrespects or demeans you, can also make you less willing to speak up for yourself or pursue ambitious goals.

Gender, race, and sexual orientation. Scores of studies show women are socialized to worry more about how they're perceived and, therefore, to take fewer risks. Racial and cultural background and sexual orientation can make a difference, too. If you've been on the receiving end of discrimination, or are a member of any marginalized identity, you may have also internalized some negative, untrue messages about your potential and whether you "belong."

MISINFORMATION

Lack of self-confidence can come from not knowing the "rules" of the confidence game. For example, if we think we have to *feel* confident in order to *act* confidently, we set ourselves up for failure. As we saw in the example of Darnell and the city council meeting, it goes the other way around.

Perfectionism is another form of faulty thinking that contributes to low self-confidence. If we believe we have to have something all figured out before we take action, those thoughts can keep us from doing the things we value. Even learning and understanding what confidence is and isn't, as you're doing in this chapter, is a big step toward boosting it.

Many media messages are designed to make us feel lacking. Companies that want to sell you products usually start by making you feel bad about yourself, often by introducing a "problem" with your body that you would never have noticed otherwise. (The movie *Mean Girls* memorably skewered this idea: The main character, new to American high school culture after years of homeschooling in Africa, is bewildered when her new clique stands around a mirror criticizing themselves. "My hairline is so weird," says one. "My nail beds suck!" proclaims another.)

Now that social media has become ubiquitous, the messages hit closer to home. It's easy to believe that everyone around you has the perfect marriage, a dream career, and supermodel looks to boot. But remember: What people post online is heavily curated and edited. Everyone has bad days, self-doubt, and physical imperfections. They just don't trot them out on Facebook!

"ONE REASON WE STRUGGLE WITH INSECURITY: WE'RE COMPARING OUR BEHIND-THE-SCENES TO EVERYONE ELSE'S HIGHLIGHT REEL."

—STEVEN FURTICK

ANXIETY AND DEPRESSION

It's common for anxiety and depression to go hand in hand with self-confidence issues. If you've already been diagnosed with an anxiety disorder or depression and are working with a therapist, you could bring in your workbook and perhaps go through it together. If you're not sure whether these issues might be affecting you, I've provided screening tools and a list of other resources in the back of the book (see page 153). It's brave of you to address your self-assurance stumbling blocks, and building confidence will also help you lessen anxiety and depression.

Which of the contributing factors described in this section resonate the most with you?

_____

_____

_____

_____

What specific experiences in your life do you think had the biggest negative effects on your self-confidence?

_____

_____

_____

_____

The Benefits of Improving Confidence

Confidence is linked to almost every element involved in a happy and fulfilling life. I'll highlight a few of the benefits of self-confidence below, and in the rest of the book, you'll learn strategies to achieve them.

LESS FEAR AND ANXIETY

The more confident you become, the more you'll be able to calm the voice inside you that says, "I can't do it." You'll be able to unhook from your thoughts and take action in line with your values.

If you've suffered from low self-confidence, you're probably familiar with rumination—the tendency to mull over worries and perceived mistakes, replaying them ad nauseam. Excessive rumination is linked to both anxiety and depression, and it can make us withdraw from the world. But by filling up your tank with confidence, or fuel for action, you'll be able to break the cycle of over-thinking and quiet your inner critic.

GREATER MOTIVATION

Building confidence means taking small steps that leave a lasting sense of accomplishment. If you've ever learned a language, mastered a skill, reached a fitness goal, or otherwise overcome setbacks to get to where you wanted to be, you're well on your way already.

You might be thinking, "Well, sure, I was proud of my A in honors calculus back in high school, but what does that have to do with anything now?" If you think back to a key accomplishment in your life, you'll likely find it took a lot of perseverance. If you could triumph through adversity then, you can do it in other areas of your life where you feel self-doubt.

As your confidence grows, you'll find yourself more driven to stretch your abilities. "What-if" thoughts will still arise: "What if I fail?" "What if I embarrass myself?" But with self-assurance, those thoughts will no longer be paralyzing. Instead, you'll be able to grin and act anyway, feeling energized by your progress in pursuing goals that mean something to you.

MORE RESILIENCE

Confidence gives you the skills and coping methods to handle setbacks and failure. Remember, self-confidence doesn't mean you won't sometimes fail. But you'll know you can handle challenges and not be crippled by them. Even when things don't turn out anywhere close to what you planned, you'll be able to avoid beating yourself up.

As you keep pushing yourself to try new things, you'll start to truly under-stand how failure and mistakes lead to growth. An acceptance that failure is part of life will start to take root. Paradoxically, by being more willing to fail, you'll actually succeed more—because you're not waiting for everything to be 100 percent perfect before you act. Taking more shots will mean making more of them.

IMPROVED RELATIONSHIPS

It might seem counterintuitive, but when you have more self-confidence, you're less focused on yourself. We've all been guilty of walking into a room and thinking, "They're all looking at me and judging me. They don't like me; they think I'm ignorant!" The truth is, people are wrapped up in their own thoughts and worries. When you get out of your own head, you'll be able to genuinely engage with others.

You'll enjoy your interactions more because you won't be so worried about the kind of impression you're making, and you won't be comparing yourself to others. Your relaxed state will put others at ease as well, helping you forge deeper connections.

Self-confidence can also breed deeper empathy. When you're fully present in the moment, you're more likely to notice that your date seems to be a little down, or that a friend in the corner of the party looks like she needs a shoulder to cry on. When you're not preoccupied with your own self-doubt, you can be the person who reaches out to help others with their problems.

STRONGER SENSE OF YOUR AUTHENTIC SELF

Finally, confidence roots you in who you really are. You'll be able to accept your weaknesses, knowing they don't change your self-worth. You'll also be able to celebrate your strengths and use them more fully.

Your actions will be in line with your principles, giving you a greater sense of purpose. You'll know who you are and what you stand for. You'll have the skills to show up, stand up, and speak up. In other words, you'll be able to let your best self shine through.

The Self-Confidence Workbook: Make It Your Own

Confidence is all about knowing yourself, and that holds true when it comes to working through this book. Color in it, underline it, doodle in it—whatever works best for you! If it would help to buy a notebook so you can jot down your thoughts as you go along, that's great. If you'd rather work through the exercises out loud with a therapist, a spouse, or a trusted friend, that works, too. It will be beneficial to read each chapter without skipping any, but feel free to disregard advice that doesn't apply to you.

Take note of information in this chapter that resonated with you the most, and let it guide you through the rest of the book. If you find yourself obsessively dwelling on negative thoughts, you might want to focus on chapter 5, which deals with improving faulty thinking patterns. If you don't spend a lot of time ruminating but are still not sure how to take steps toward the goals that scare you the most, chapter 7 might hold the best tools for you. The Self-Confidence Scale in the next section can also help you figure out what to concentrate on.

Progress through the book at your own pace, and do the exercises in whatever setting is most comfortable for you, whether that's a quiet neighborhood park or a room in your house where you can blast your favorite music. Yes, this is a "work" book, but you can also play with it and make it fun.

The Self-Confidence Scale

Now that you have a better understanding of what self-confidence is, what it isn't, and why it matters, let's determine your starting point. Read each statement on the following page and circle A if it is true for you most of the time, B if it is true for you some of the time, and C if it is not usually true.

I have a realistic sense of my strengths and weaknesses.	A B C
I am willing to take risks for something I believe in.	A B C
I plan and prepare for new experiences.	A B C
I have ways to cope with fear and doubt.	A B C
I take time to remember my past successes.	A B C
I recognize failure as a part of life.	A B C
I can cope with unexpected changes.	A B C
I am comfortable asking for help and support.	A B C
I know what I value in life.	A B C
My actions generally line up with my values.	A B C
I don't give up easily.	A B C
I realize not everyone will like or approve of me.	A B C
I have a sense of my inherent worth.	A B C
I understand setbacks are normal and to be expected.	A B C
I don't beat up on myself when I'm going through a rough time.	A B C
My thoughts don't paralyze me when trying something new.	A B C

Here's how to interpret your score:

Mostly As: You're doing a great job of not allowing obstacles to get in your way of meeting valued goals. This book will help you learn new skills to improve your confidence even more.

Mostly Bs: You're right in the middle, sometimes recognizing your accomplishments and other times focusing on where you're falling short. Your answers indicate you may fall prey to common pitfalls that undermine self-confidence. This book will help you identify those areas so you can more consistently enjoy self-confidence.

Mostly Cs: Your self-confidence is a little shaky, but that's okay. Remember, there is no one with total self-confidence all of the time. The tools in this book will help you ease up on yourself, notice your accomplishments, and find ways to handle setbacks. You'll learn, step-by-step, how to set goals that mean something to you, how to meet those goals, and how to cope with fear along the way.

Use the space below to note any thoughts or feelings you might have after taking this quiz. Take note of any particular items you'd like to focus on as you move through the book. Remember to give yourself credit for embarking on this journey.

CONSIDER YOUR STRENGTHS

No matter how down you feel, remember to recognize your talents and good qualities. Try making a list of your strengths and referring back to it when you feel yourself focusing on your perceived flaws or mistakes.

Think back on compliments from other people. What have they told you about yourself that you otherwise might not notice or acknowledge?

Remember past accomplishments. It can be something other people recognized, like being at the top of your class, or something only you know about, like a quiet act of service to make life easier for someone else. List any accomplishments that come to mind.

Think about the qualities you try to cultivate. No one's perfect, but if you're actively trying to be an honorable, good person, give yourself some credit and list some of these qualities below.

Chapter Takeaways

Now you have a clear vision of confidence: what it is, what it's not, and how attainable it is for anyone willing to pursue it. (If you're interested, you can learn a little more about yourself and participate in research on self-confidence by taking the online Confidence Code Assessment at http://theconfidencecode .com/confidence-quiz.)

The next chapter is all about where you're going. You'll be setting goals for yourself and learning about the tools that will help you get there.

Action Items

Here are some specific actions you can take to implement the lessons and ideas you learned in this chapter:

1. Write down a favorite confidence quote and put it somewhere you'll see it often.
2. Consider sharing with someone you trust that you're reading this book. I bet you'll find you're not alone in your desire for more confidence.
3. Do you have a photograph of a time you felt confident and successful? It could be a graduation photo, a picture of you as a kid after you learned to ride a bike, or anything else that resonates with you. Hang it on your fridge or bathroom mirror, and reflect on the steps it took to get to that point.
4. Watch a YouTube video of someone you admire who exudes confidence.
5. Try taking a break from social media for a day or even a week. See whether the urge to compare yourself with others starts to subside a little.

CHAPTER 2:

SETTING GOALS AND GETTING STARTED

• •

"THE SCARIEST MOMENT IS ALWAYS JUST BEFORE YOU START."

—STEPHEN KING

Nia had lacked self-confidence for so long, she wasn't even sure what she really wanted anymore.

She had been single for more than five years. Even though she'd always imagined herself as a wife and mother, she had convinced herself that maybe it just wasn't going to happen. The fear of going on dates and being rejected had become so strong that she had stopped trying altogether.

Avoiding the stresses of dating felt rewarding in the short term: After all, Nia didn't have to experience the overwhelming fear of embarrassing herself or somehow not measuring up. But when she envisioned a world in which she had unlimited self-confidence, she knew immediately it would include a romantic life of flirting, dating, and ultimately, building nurturing relationships.

Nia decided to set small goals to expose herself to her fear. She would make a profile on a dating app and ask her friends from church if they knew anyone to set her up with. As she took these steps, her confidence grew, and soon she found herself going on dates and even enjoying them. Sometimes the dates were awkward, or just bad—and that was okay, too. Nia knew that by pursuing her goals, she was starting to live the life she really wanted.

As you learned in chapter 1, confidence is all about action. If taking action in the face of fear, doubt, or lack of motivation were easy, our real lives might look more like our wildest dreams. Fortunately, there are many strategies you can use to increase your self-confidence, and you'll get a taste of them in this chapter.

First, you'll think about what you really value and want in life: Where do you hope confidence will take you? You'll set goals to get you there.

Then I'll walk you through the strategies you'll be exploring in the rest of the book. You'll learn to examine and reframe your negative thoughts, commit to taking positive actions, expose yourself to your fears in small doses, and increase mindfulness to find a greater sense of calm.

The Importance of Goals

By now, you may have realized you're feeling confident in some areas of your life but not so confident in others. Whatever the case, you need goals, or your efforts will lack focus and direction.

What do you want to accomplish? You might feel the answer is obvious: "I want to be more self-confident." Although this is a desirable goal, it's too general to serve as a helpful road map for action.

One way to think about your goals is to ask yourself some questions:

What opportunities have I turned down because I didn't feel confident enough?

What opportunities would I pursue if I had more confidence?

Are there activities I've avoided because of lack of confidence?

Another way to think about lack of self-confidence is fear. Ask yourself, "In what ways have I limited my life because of fear?"

Now you're a little more prepared to come up with some goals that are specific, realistic, and consistent with your values.

SPECIFIC

Once you have a general aim in mind, it's important to come up with goals that paint a picture of what success will look like. These goals should be measurable, so that you'll know when you're achieving them and when you need more practice. Here's an example:

Aim:
I want to be more socially confident at my new job.

Goals:
I will be less anxious when introduced to a coworker.
I will be able to make eye contact.
I won't turn down invitations to have lunch with someone.
I will be able to carry on a brief conversation in the break room.
I will stop assuming I'm saying the wrong thing all the time.

REALISTIC

Goals also need to be realistic. For example, you can't expect to give a flawless speech or proceed through life never feeling nervous. Your goals should not demand perfection, because that sets you up for failure.

That's not to say you should give in to self-doubt. By all means, dream big as you're writing your goals—you'll learn how to break them into bite-size, doable pieces. But remember that you're only human.

Reality can also force us to change our goals as we go on. For instance, a devastating injury could stop you from pursuing a job you really wanted or force you to put off starting a family. Giving up on goals can be incredibly painful. But nothing will be able to stop you from living your values and making new goals that take into account your changed life circumstances.

Values are the principles that give our lives meaning and allow us to persevere through adversity. But often, our lives don't perfectly align with our values, particularly when a lack of self-confidence stands in the way.

Sometimes it takes reflection to know which values you really hold closest to your heart. Here are some questions to help you get started.

What is important to you? Try to distinguish between what other people think you should care about and what you truly value.

What sort of person do you want to be at work? In your relationships? In your community?

If you could wave a magic wand and have your ideal life, what would it look like?

Now, review the list of commonly held values on the next page. Circle the three values that resonate the most with you.

It might be hard to pick just three, and that's okay. Some items on the list could be combined—for instance, loyalty and openness might fold into your core value of friendship. If you have to pick more than three, try to keep your total below six so that your list doesn't get too unwieldy.

Acceptance	Faith	Optimism
Accomplishment	Family	Originality
Altruism	Freedom	Patience
Artistic Nature	Friendship	Peace
Awareness	Generosity	Persistence
Beauty	Gratitude	Personal Growth
Bravery	Growth	Play
Calm	Happiness	Practicality
Carefulness	Harmony	Productivity
Commitment	Health	Reason
Community	Honesty	Reliability
Compassion	Humility	Resourcefulness
Confidence	Humor	Risk
Contentment	Individuality	Security
Connection	Intuitiveness	Service
Creativity	Joy	Silence
Curiosity	Justice	Simplicity
Dependability	Kindness	Skillfulness
Dignity	Knowledge	Spirituality
Discipline	Leadership	Spontaneity
Empathy	Learning	Stability
Energy	Love	Strength
Enthusiasm	Loyalty	Thoughtfulness
Equality	Mastery	Understanding
Ethicality	Maturity	Uniqueness
Excellence	Meaning	Trustworthiness
Excitement	Mindfulness	Truth
Expressive	Nature	Welcoming Spirit
Fairness	Openness	Wisdom

Once you've chosen your top three core values, pick one and spend about 10 minutes writing about what it means to you. Explore why that value is important to you and how you express it in your everyday life.

MINI CONFIDENCE BOOSTERS

This book's goal is, of course, to help you build your self-confidence over the long term. But that doesn't mean you can't make use of quick "hype-up" strategies ahead of a big day. Here are some ideas.

A favorite outfit: If you have an outfit that makes you feel like a million bucks, by all means, wear it when you're facing your biggest confidence challenges. Oddly, this works even if you're going into a phone interview where no one will see you.

A playlist: Listening to your favorite confidence-boosting anthems can be a big help as you're going through your morning routine on a stressful day. It's a bonus if they make you want to dance around your bathroom and sing along, working through those nerves!

A reward: If you're trying to push yourself to do something scary, it can help to promise yourself a little reward: "If I ask José on a date, I'll buy myself an ice cream cone afterward." If you tie the reward to your effort rather than the outcome, it will remind you that action itself is more important than success.

A role model: Picture someone you know who comes off as confident but not arrogant or pushy. You'll often find you can emulate that person's fearlessness for a moment.

A confidence buddy: Telling a friend ahead of time that you're committing to taking a certain step will help ensure that you do it. I'll talk more about this strategy later in the book.

Setting Your Goals

Keeping your core values top of mind is essential to setting meaningful goals, as I saw with one of my clients years ago.

Jamal came to me for general anxiety concerns. He tended to second-guess himself a lot and become caught up in a worry cycle. He also didn't have a lot of confidence in his abilities, particularly at work.

During one session, Jamal told me that he had been offered a promotion. The new role would involve leading small teams of people and occasionally speaking to large groups. It would also involve some travel.

Initially, I assumed that Jamal would want the position if not for his insecurities. After discussing the requirements of the new job with me, Jamal agreed that with some encouragement and practice, he would be able to fulfill the duties. However, he also brought up that the new position would require many more hours of working, and he'd be out of town more often.

He had a family to consider: his wife, their five-year-old, and a new baby. Although Jamal certainly valued career advancement, spending time with his family was actually more important. Jamal ended up turning down the promotion, but not out of fear and insecurity. He turned it down because he was rooted in the knowledge that he was acting in line with his values.

No one can tell you what is most important to you. Sure, our culture will say that having a better job, a bigger house, and a fancier car is what we need to make us happy. It takes a lot of strength and conviction to not just go along with societal expectations. Self-confidence doesn't always look like the "big" move. It can be the confidence to say, "No, this opportunity is not right for me at this time."

"WHAT YOU GET BY REACHING YOUR GOALS IS NOT NEARLY SO IMPORTANT AS WHAT YOU BECOME BY REACHING THEM."

—ZIG ZIGLAR

Now it's your turn. Below are some categories in which you might want to consider self-confidence goals. Take some time to think about them and make notes in the space provided.

I don't want you to become overwhelmed. You might have goals in each of the areas listed, or you might want to select just one area to work on for now. Follow the steps in this book and then come back to the other areas. What you'll likely find is that when you gain confidence in one area, it will spill over to the others.

RELATIONSHIPS

If you had the confidence to fully live your values in your relationships with family and friends, what would you be doing? Would you approach conflict differently? Would you set stronger boundaries? What about your love life—what would you do if you had unlimited confidence? Set some specific, realistic, and values-driven goals below.

PARENTING

If you had the confidence to fully live your values as a parent, what would you be doing? Would you participate differently in your children's lives or model differently for them? Would you take a different approach to discipline? Set some specific, realistic, and values-driven goals below.

FAMILY

If you had the confidence to fully live your values in your relationships with your parents, siblings, and other family members, what would you be doing? Set some specific, realistic, and values-driven goals below.

_____

_____

_____

_____

WORK

If you had the confidence to fully live your values in your career, what kind of work would you be doing? What would your role be within an organization? How would you relate to coworkers? What kinds of opportunities would you accept? Set some specific, realistic, and values-driven goals below.

_____

_____

_____

_____

COMMUNITY

If you had the confidence to fully live your values in your community, what would you be doing? What causes or organizations would you be involved in, and what would your role be? How would you connect with others and make a difference in the ways that are most meaningful to you? Set some specific, realistic, and values-driven goals below.

HEALTH

If you had the confidence to fully live your values when it comes to your physical and mental well-being, what would you be doing? Would you join a gym or exercise class, regardless of what people might think? Would you get back to an old hobby or activity that always helped you deal with stress, even if maybe you aren't as "good" at it anymore? Set some specific, realistic, and values-driven goals below.

LIFE ENJOYMENT

Are there other ways in which you're holding yourself back from enjoying life because of a lack of self-confidence? For instance, maybe you avoid going to the beach because you don't like how you look in a swimsuit, or you don't celebrate your own birthday because you don't want to draw attention to yourself. If there are things you'd genuinely like to do but haven't found the confidence for, write them in the form of specific, realistic, and values-driven goals below.

Tools for the Journey

Now that you've set some goals for yourself, let's talk about the tools you'll be using to get there. The concepts and exercises detailed in this book are based on evidence-based therapies, meaning they've been shown to work in rigorous research studies. Although the types of therapy described below have some differences, they complement each other nicely. Therapists often combine strategies from these various approaches, and tools from different therapies will be woven throughout this book.

It's possible that not every single strategy will work for you, and that's okay. Some people will naturally embrace and get more out of one type of treatment over another. That's why I'm detailing a wide range of strategies so you can tailor a plan that works for you.

COGNITIVE BEHAVIORAL THERAPY (CBT)

If you've read other psychology or self-help books, you've likely heard of CBT, as it's one of the most widely used types of treatment for depression, anxiety, and many other conditions. Psychologist Albert Ellis was one of the first to devise therapeutic techniques aimed at changing thoughts that lead to unnecessary distress. Psychiatrist Aaron Beck also showed how the roots of depression can often be identified as irrational thoughts. These two men are often cited as the fathers of cognitive therapy, now known as Cognitive Behavioral Therapy.

WHY IT WORKS

The approaches in this book have been shown to work in clinical settings—but they're also well suited to learning on your own.

All of these therapies share common characteristics:	What this means for you:
Supported by research	You know it works
Focused on the here-and-now	No blaming your parents
Often organized into steps	Easy to understand
Designed for everyday situations	Applies to your life
Practical skills	Simple to put into practice
Typically short-term focus	Quicker results

Let's look at one principle of CBT in action. Imagine you're walking down the street and you see someone on the other side walking toward you. You get a little closer and recognize the person as someone you know from your Zumba class. You look up, smile, wave, and shout, "Hi!" The other person keeps walking and doesn't acknowledge you. There are many ways you could interpret this situation. What would you say to yourself? Circle A, B, or C.

A   She must not like me. I'm such a loser.
B   She must not have seen me.
C   She's so stuck up. I can't believe she didn't say hi.

Now, imagine how you'd feel in each case.

If you thought to yourself, "She must not like me," you'd likely feel sad, embarrassed, or something along those lines.

If you thought to yourself, "She must not have seen me," you'd likely feel neutral, or maybe simply a little disappointed.

If you circled C, you might feel angry.

Notice that the event is the same. The only thing that has changed is your interpretation of the situation, or what you're saying to yourself. The principle behind CBT is that self-talk matters.

Now think about a time you came out of a situation feeling less confident, and fill out the diagram below.

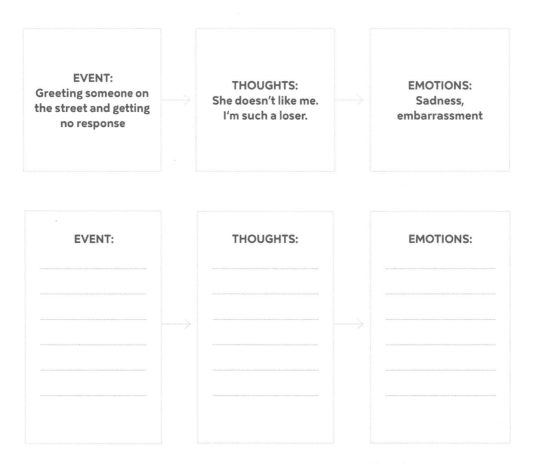

EVENT:
Greeting someone on the street and getting no response

THOUGHTS:
She doesn't like me.
I'm such a loser.

EMOTIONS:
Sadness, embarrassment

EVENT:

THOUGHTS:

EMOTIONS:

So what does this have to do with confidence? Low self-confidence is often based upon unhelpful or untrue interpretations of a situation. If you believe your Zumba classmate didn't wave at you because you're a loser, you're much less likely to risk saying hi or starting a conversation with her in the future. That's why CBT, a set of methods to identify such thoughts and reframe them, is often so useful in building self-assurance.

In chapter 5, you'll learn to notice distorted thinking, such as: "I always make a fool of myself when I try to speak up in a meeting." Once you can catch yourself having those thoughts, you can break them down: Does this thought really reflect reality? Is it effective in getting you closer to your goals? Then, in chapter 6, you'll learn how your thoughts combine and interact to form belief systems. Everyone has these core belief systems, but we're often not aware of the power they can exert on our behavior. I'll provide exercises to help you bring both your thoughts and beliefs out into the light, so they won't keep you from reaching your self-confidence goals.

You'll learn to envision likelier outcomes and realize that even in the worst-case scenario, you'd be able to dust yourself off and move on. You'll also begin to give yourself more credit for the positive things you do instead of beating yourself up over perceived mistakes. These mind-set changes are meant to spur you ahead to action, the cornerstone of confidence.

ACCEPTANCE AND COMMITMENT THERAPY (ACT)

ACT (pronounced like the word *act*) was developed in 1986 by Steven C. Hayes, a professor in the psychology department at the University of Nevada. Hayes took a somewhat controversial view, at least in terms of mainstream psychology at the time, asserting that suffering is an inevitable and essential part of being human. He argued that accepting this suffering, rather than running from it, was a more effective way to build a meaningful life.

He also took a different view of thoughts than his CBT colleagues. Recall that in CBT you aim to notice your negative thoughts so that you can replace them with more helpful ones. ACT doesn't place as much emphasis on the content of your thoughts. At the heart of ACT is the idea that you can learn to live with even unpleasant thoughts, as long as you don't give them power over your actions.

ACT teaches you not to avoid worry, fear, or doubt, because negative feelings are just a natural part of life. Struggling against your anxiety can often make it worse, as you'll recognize if you've ever thought, "Why am I so nervous? What's the matter with me?"

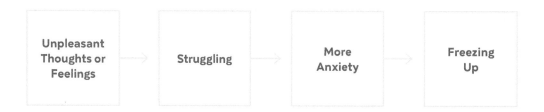

When you find yourself thinking, "I can't do this," or "This is going to be a disaster," you can learn to notice the thought and let it pass you by without deciding it's the gospel truth. Detaching from your negative thoughts helps prevent rumination, which is linked to anxiety and depression, and lessens the urge to run from discomfort by indulging in harmful behaviors such as binge drinking or overeating.

You may not be able to evict your inner critic from your mind, but you can learn to tune out its relentless negativity and move forward—or "act"—with confidence.

ACT has a lot to offer, and I'll be making use of many of its components throughout the book. Remember, too, how I said these schools of therapy can complement each other. Although anxiety and "negative" thinking are not dangerous, I don't see anything wrong with learning some ways to be more comfortable. In chapter 4, I'll show you some techniques to calm your body, and in chapter 5, I'll show you some ways to calm your mind. Your anxiety won't completely go away, but it will likely lessen over time.

"STAY AFRAID, BUT DO IT ANYWAY. WHAT'S IMPORTANT IS THE ACTION. YOU DON'T HAVE TO WAIT TO BE CONFIDENT. JUST DO IT AND EVENTUALLY THE CONFIDENCE WILL FOLLOW."

—CARRIE FISHER

EXPOSURE THERAPY

Exposure therapy sometimes falls under the umbrella of CBT, as it is a behavioral therapy aimed at helping people overcome anxiety and fear.

You may have heard about the work of psychologist Edna Foa, who uses exposure therapy to treat post-traumatic stress disorder. In 2010, *Time* named her one of the most influential people in the world. Foa helps people identify thoughts and situations that trigger the most fear and then gently exposes sufferers to them. She and others have shown that exposure therapy works well in many situations, from spider phobias to stage fright—and it can help you develop your confidence, too.

You already know avoiding all forms of discomfort is not a path to a happy, fulfilling life. But that doesn't mean you're itching to step out your front door and go give a public speech, ask someone on a date, or do whatever scares you the most.

Don't worry—I'm not going to ask you to dive into the deep end and learn to swim! Research shows that being forced to face a big fear all at once only leaves you traumatized, swearing you'll never try again.

Exposure therapy is more like dipping your toes in the water. You start with a tiny first step that scares you just a little bit, getting used to the fear and realizing you're capable of handling it. Then you build up gradually to bigger and bigger steps, until you're finally swimming in the pool.

Some exposure therapy is done in real life. For example, I took a client who was afraid of heights to a nearby building for several sessions, working our way up the floors until she was comfortable standing close to a railing many stories up. Other times, imagining the situation is enough to practice grappling with the fear.

The key is repetition; you can't try facing your fear once and then wait a year and try again. Here's an example of how Kurt, who feels he doesn't have the confidence to attend networking events in his industry, might use exposure therapy to overcome that fear.

Week 1: Kurt will go to a networking event with someone he already knows and stay just 30 minutes.

Week 2: He will attend an event with someone he knows and introduce himself to at least one new person.

Week 3: Kurt will go to an event with someone he knows and introduce himself to three new people.

Week 4: Kurt will go to an event by himself, greet everyone he's met before, and introduce himself to three new people.

Week 5: He will go to an event by himself, introduce himself to five new people, and follow up with one of them via email the next day to set up a one-on-one coffee meeting.

I'll talk more about how to make your own exposure goals in chapter 7. For now, think about something you usually avoid. What is a small step you could take to move you in the desired direction? Now, try to break that step into an even smaller step. I want you to get in the habit of thinking in baby steps. You'll be much more likely to follow through if it doesn't seem that far out of your norm.

MINDFULNESS-BASED THERAPIES

The final type of therapeutic approach I'll draw from is that of mindfulness-based therapies. Adding mindfulness into the mix of cognitive and behavioral approaches has gained wide acceptance and popularity over the past decade. But even as early as the 1970s, Jon Kabat-Zinn had integrated principles of mindfulness into his work with medical patients. He is the founder of the mindfulness-based stress reduction program (MBSR), which has helped millions of people with heart disease, chronic pain, and other health problems achieve improvement in symptoms and greater wellness overall. Now MBSR is used in nonmedical settings, such as businesses, and there are even MBSR programs for adolescents. In the late 1980s, psychologist Marsha Linehan created dialectical behavior therapy, which added the concept of acceptance to mindfulness. (You'll learn about acceptance in chapter 3.)

So what is mindfulness? Mindfulness is intentionally paying attention to the present moment with an attitude of openness and curiosity. There's also a spirit of nonjudgment to this process. I know this may sound abstract at this point. Don't worry. It's not as "woo woo" as it might sound, and later, I'll break it down into easy steps.

One benefit of mindfulness is that it's a helpful way of disconnecting from the onslaught of negativity from your inner critic by reconnecting with the world around you. Although our minds will always tend to draw us into worries and what-ifs, it's possible to train yourself to come back to Earth when you find your-self getting sucked into a ruminative spiral.

TRY, TRY AGAIN

Failure is a fact of life—and a useful one, too. If you cruise through life avoiding risks, you'll likely never learn or grow in any meaningful way. Even the most confident people experience self-doubt, but what matters is that they forge ahead anyway, not allowing their fear to increase through inaction.

When what you're aiming for is progress, it's easy to forget that failure is not pushing you backward. Mistakes don't halt your momentum; they help you figure out a better path.

As you try to build self-confidence, you're going to have some days when things just don't go right. Maybe you'll try to speak up in a meeting, but your thoughts will come out jumbled and cause an awkward pause. Or maybe you'll try to set firmer rules with your children, and they'll stick out their tongues and keep misbehaving. The most important thing is to get back on the proverbial horse and try again.

Try this the next time you're facing a failure: Ask yourself, What did I do that worked? What did I do that didn't work? What can I do differently next time? If you're stuck, seek feedback from someone you trust about how to improve.

Getting comfortable with failure is how you ultimately let go of perfectionism, get messy, and make mistakes, until eventually you find a way that works. There's no better feeling than knowing that you earned success through your own hard work. *That's* confidence.

In chapter 4, I'll walk you through mindfulness exercises that will help lower your anxiety levels, helping you to face your biggest confidence challenges. For now, here's one of the simplest ways to start: Focus on your breath.

- Notice the rhythm and sensation of your breathing. If you're like 99.9 percent of people, your mind will stray. You'll start thinking about your to-do list, wondering if you're doing this right, thinking about what you're going to have for lunch . . . All of that is completely normal and does not mean you're not doing it properly.
- When you notice that your mind has strayed, gently bring your focus back to the breath. The key is to be gentle. You don't say, "I'm so bad at this." Just think, "Oh, there goes my mind wandering. That's okay. I'll just return my attention to the breath."
- After a few minutes of practice, you'll likely find that you're a little calmer and less distracted.

Chapter Takeaways

Now you know the science. Scores of people have improved their self-confidence using the methods you're about to learn in part 2. You might still be a little wary, but I hope you're also willing to give it a try. When you feel scared or intimidated, you can always come back to the values and goals you listed and remind yourself that the efforts you're making are leading you to a better, fuller life. In the next part of the book, you'll start practicing these strategies, starting with accepting yourself.

Here are some specific actions you can take to implement the lessons and ideas you learned in this chapter:

1. In the coming days, take note of any events that put a dent in your confidence, and write down what thoughts you had interpreting those events. (You can carry around a notebook or keep a note in your smartphone for this exercise.)
2. Practice noticing your breathing for a few minutes each day without trying to change anything. Where do you feel the breath? Do you feel the air at your nostrils? Do you notice the movement of your chest and abdomen?
3. Pick a "mini confidence booster" (see page 29) and try it out.
4. Watch Joe Kowan's charming TED Talk, "How I Beat Stage Fright."
5. Write down your top three values on a slip of paper and put it in a place you'll see it every day.

PART 2

THE STRATEGIES

Now that you have a clear vision of what you would do with more self-confidence, let's talk about how to get there. Part 2 will give you practical, accessible strategies for building self-confidence across different areas of your life.

Using tools from the therapies you learned about in part 1, you'll start learning to diminish your anxiety around intimidating situations. You'll practice accepting yourself and what's going on in your life rather than fighting against or avoiding unpleasant feelings. You'll get in the habit of speaking to yourself with self-compassion, recognizing what went right instead of beating yourself up for every little mistake.

Instead of trying to shrink or disappear when you're nervous, you'll learn to breathe deeply, take up space, and take your time. Mindfulness techniques will help you stop the runaway train of rumination and see the world that's right in front of you. You'll also learn to recognize unhelpful thought patterns and core beliefs, and redirect yourself toward more useful ones. You'll get comfortable with your inner critic as a passenger in your head, noticing your inevitable moments of self-doubt but not letting them change your course of action.

Most importantly, you'll take steps toward your goals, leaving your mind and stepping out into the real world, where confidence takes root. If you're starting to worry or wondering if any of this will really help you, that's normal. All I ask is that you give it a try—make a good-faith effort here, and you'll see that it pays dividends. I'll be cheering you along every step of the way.

CHAPTER 3

PRACTICE ACCEPTANCE

· · · · · · · · · · · · ·

"THE CURIOUS PARADOX IS THAT WHEN I ACCEPT MYSELF JUST AS I AM, THEN I CAN CHANGE."

—CARL ROGERS

At first, acceptance is a difficult concept to grasp. After all, you bought this book because you want to change. Hearing that you should practice acceptance might make you think you're being told to settle for the way things are and not bother to try to improve them. But once you understand what acceptance really means, it will make a huge difference in how you proceed—not only in your quest for more confidence but for your life in general.

The best way to understand acceptance is to think about an equation often cited in the psychology world: Suffering = Pain X Resistance.

Imagine you're stuck in a traffic jam and you're going to be late for an important meeting. The pain is real: You hate being late, and there's nothing you can do about it. The resistance part kicks in when your self-talk starts: "I shouldn't be caught in traffic. This is horrible. What is going on? Is there an accident up ahead?" Your resistance amplifies the pain and creates the suffering.

Once you're at the meeting, you're about to give a brief project update and your stomach starts to churn. Your mind starts up: "I can't believe this is happening again. Why can't I be like normal people and just be able to participate in a simple meeting without getting so anxious?" Again, the pain is the experience of your stomach hurting. Resisting it is what makes you panicked, unfocused, and more likely to make mistakes during the presentation.

We often can't control the pain part of the equation. Life happens. What we can usually control is our reaction to it. By not piling on to the pain with resistance, we'll have less suffering.

The antidote to resistance is acceptance.

- Acceptance is a willingness to see reality without judgment.
- Acceptance does not equal approval.
- Acceptance does not mean you won't take appropriate action.
- Acceptance isn't putting up with misery.
- Acceptance is the starting point for change.

The first step toward developing lasting self-confidence is to practice acceptance—of your strengths, your weaknesses, and yourself. I'll show you how.

Revisit Your Goals

Now that you understand what acceptance is, think about how it applies to your own life. Specifically, refer back to the goals you set in the previous chapter and write down a few thoughts about how learning to practice acceptance might help you achieve them. For instance, maybe you've recently experienced a setback to your confidence, such as losing your job. It's understandable that you'd spend time mulling over the pain of what happened. But by accepting the situation as best you can, you can turn your attention to seeking new opportunities.

YOU DON'T NEED TO BE FIXED

I've been into self-improvement my whole life. At age 10, I was reading a copy of *The Power of Positive Thinking* by Norman Vincent Peale that I found on my grandmother's bookshelf. Later, I spent hours browsing the self-help section at bookstores and libraries, trying to find that one book that would make me feel "good enough." Before Pinterest, I made my own notebooks of inspirational quotes. I started a blog called *The Self-Compassion Project*, only to realize that self-compassion is not a project; it's a practice and a process.

It took me many decades to learn I am not a broken human being; I am fine just as I am. Sure, I set goals and try to learn and grow in areas that I value. But now, I do so from a position of self-acceptance and a sense of worthiness that doesn't come from external sources.

So it's a bit paradoxical for me to be writing this workbook. I want to (and will) offer you strategies and tools that I know truly work to build confidence. As you learned in chapter 1, self-confidence offers many benefits. But I also want to balance this with my deep belief that you are not a problem to be solved, and you certainly don't need to be "fixed." My hope is that by the end of this book, you'll share my belief.

Take a moment to reflect on how acceptance might help you pursue your goals.

Accept Your Strengths

Lydia finds herself greeting even her biggest blessings in life with the same troubling thought: "What's the catch?" When she wins a big contest in her industry, she thinks, "Well, there must not have been many entries this year." When a man she likes asks her on a date, she works herself into a frenzy—she's sure he's made a mistake, and she'll soon be revealed as the big dork she is. When someone gives her a compliment, she always deflects, giving the credit to somebody else.

If you've battled low self-confidence, Lydia might sound a lot like you. Resistance doesn't come only when we face pain in life. Many of us resist compliments and good fortune, too, because we just don't think we deserve them. Women in particular are often averse to acknowledging their strengths, believing they'll be guilty of braggadocio or seem egotistical if they do.

But accepting your strengths isn't about building yourself up in comparison to others. You don't need to tell yourself you're the *best* salesperson, parent, or point guard in the local recreational basketball league. Instead, you're trying to reduce the suffering in your life by decreasing resistance.

When you've worked hard, give yourself credit. When you do a good job or try something new, let yourself feel some pride. Accepting your strengths helps you keep your weaknesses in perspective, one of the keys to walking through the world with confidence.

IDENTIFY YOUR STRENGTHS

To get started, jot down some notes responding to the prompts in the following worksheet.

Compliments I've received:	Challenges I've overcome:	An important role I've fulfilled:

An important task I've tackled:	Skills I enjoy using regardless of the task:	A time I've helped someone else:

When you're done, read over what you've written and try to notice themes.

List three or more of your strengths below.

WHY WE FIGHT ACCEPTING OUR STRENGTHS

Many people are brought up to believe that accepting our strengths means being prideful. We don't want to boast or come off to others as "holier-than-thou." Maybe you know there's something you're good at, but you truly don't think it's a big deal, often thinking that anyone could do it if they really tried.

There are other reasons you might bristle at the idea of noticing your own strong points. "If I tell myself I'm already doing well, I'll think it's okay to rest on my laurels," you might think. "I won't push myself to keep getting better." Or maybe it's hard for you to recognize your strengths as valuable because they don't fit into the norms of the world you're in. For instance, maybe you work in a dog-eat-dog corporate environment and don't see your patience and listening skills as useful—after all, you don't hear many colleagues being praised for their quiet fortitude.

All of this is natural. I'm not asking you to hold a parade for yourself, proclaiming that you're the best, or to tell yourself you're perfect and could never improve. Remember, confidence isn't the same as arrogance. It's the knowledge that you can continue to act in line with your values, no matter what life throws at you. Most of the time, that knowledge is something you can carry with you without telling anyone else, "Hey, here's what makes me so great." But sometimes you will have to advocate for yourself to reach valued goals, such as earning a promotion, and you can't do that without accepting your strengths.

CELEBRATE YOUR STRENGTHS

It's easy to feel like you're never doing enough. When you start comparing yourself to others, you might worry you're not spending enough time with your kids, staying healthy enough, or climbing the career ladder enough. Enough with "enough"! It's important to take time to celebrate everything you're doing right. This could mean unwinding with a significant other and trading stories of the day's small victories, or it could mean keeping a journal where you give yourself credit for the steps you took toward your goals.

It's also okay to bask in your accomplishments, even if it's just for an instant. If you're someone who struggles to accept others' kind words, practice saying a simple "thank you" the next time someone pays you a compliment. Not only will you feel better, but you'll make others feel good, too, by not dismissing them when they make an effort to recognize your strengths.

Accept Your Weaknesses and Imperfections

Everyone has weaknesses. They fall into different categories: There are weaknesses that have nothing to do with what matters to you in life, and others that do. There are weaknesses that stem from a lack of information or training, and there are weaknesses that stem from a lack of practice. To an extent, some weaknesses are attributable to your temperament or natural talents. What matters the most in all of these cases is how you play the hand you were dealt.

As you now know, resistance increases your suffering. If you avoid public speaking because you're terrible at it, even though it's part of a valued goal, your short-term relief is costing you the long-term satisfaction of growth and advancement. Facing the possibility of failure can be petrifying, and you might feel there's no point in trying to improve. But accepting the weakness can help make it feel less like a shameful flaw and more of an opportunity to learn and stretch yourself.

You can probably think of many weaknesses you have that really don't matter very much in terms of living your values—but for some reason, you're still bothered by them. In those situations, letting go of the shame and owning the fact that you're not perfect can be quite freeing. If you admit your weaknesses, you might be surprised how patient and helpful people can become. For instance, say you're a passionate and knowledgeable teacher, but sometimes you struggle with the technology you need to run your class. If you admit you need help, maybe with some self-deprecating humor, your students will probably step up and get things running in no time.

To get started, jot down some notes following the prompts in the worksheet below.

Recognizing Challenges

Weaknesses I'm aware of:	What's most likely to make me give up?	What trips me up time and time again?

What keeps me from moving forward?	Feedback I've received that may indicate a weakness:	What roles do I avoid?

When you're done, read over what you've written and try to notice themes.

List three or more of your challenges or weaknesses below.

_____

_____

_____

_____

_____

> *"IMPERFECTIONS ARE NOT INADEQUACIES; THEY ARE REMINDERS THAT WE'RE ALL IN THIS TOGETHER."*
>
> —BRENÉ BROWN

One of the hardest things about accepting your weaknesses is being okay with the idea that other people might see them. Sometimes we live in fear that if others *really* saw us—our struggles, our mistakes, our failures—they would reject us altogether.

But research shows the opposite is true. Vulnerability is how you connect to others. When people see that you're worried, scared, messy, or flawed, they tend to feel great relief and let you know that they are, too.

Being comfortable with imperfection doesn't mean you have to reveal every personal challenge to everyone in your life. But if you perceive a flaw in yourself that causes you great shame, consider sharing it with someone you trust. You'll likely find that the ability to live your life with authenticity takes a huge weight off your shoulders and brings you closer to those around you.

BRAIN SCIENCE 101

Our brains evolved with the primary goal of keeping us safe. In prehistoric times, this meant keeping up with the pack. Veering off by ourselves meant certain death. We're wired to notice how we differ from others and to adjust our behavior accordingly.

What this means: It's natural that we worry what others think about us. Comparisons are normal, although not often helpful.

Deep within our brain lies a complex fear network. We're programmed to register fear—and to act on it. This is the fight-or-flight response. Nature's biggest concern is our safety and survival, not whether we're enjoying ourselves in the process.

What this means: We're more likely to focus on negative aspects of ourselves and our situations. We must learn to consciously override the "negativity bias" of the brain.

Our bodies also have a mammalian part of the brain, which, when activated, leads to a "tend-and-befriend" response. For example, mammals' young are designed to attach closely with the mother to stay safe. In addition, mammals respond to a warm, soft touch and a soothing voice.

What this means: By tapping into this part of the brain, you're likely to experience less stress, both emotionally and physically. You'll learn how to do that later in this chapter.

ADOPT A GROWTH MIND-SET

Read each statement and circle the letter for the one that resonates most.

A   Either I'm good at something or I'm not.
B   I can learn to do something if I want to.

A   I tend to take feedback personally.
B   I tend to take feedback as information about how to improve.

A   When things aren't going well, I throw in the towel.

B   When things aren't going well, I see it as a challenge.

A   I stick to what I know.

B   I'm open to learning new things.

If you answered mostly *As*, you likely have what psychologist Carol Dweck terms a *fixed mind-set*. You see your traits and capabilities as more or less predetermined and set in stone. You'll hear people referring to fixed mind-sets in casual conversation—for example: "She is a natural comedian." If you answered mostly *Bs*, you have what Dweck calls a *growth mind-set*. You believe that effort and attitude play an important role in what you can accomplish.

If you identify yourself as having a fixed mind-set, don't worry. Many of us start out that way. But fortunately, even your mind-set toward change can change! Simply learning about these mind-sets can often be enough to nudge you to risk trying new things.

Look back over your challenge areas. Is there anything you might be able to learn more about through research, speaking to someone, or taking a class? Let yourself mull it over without feeling pressure to do anything just yet.

Also, tune in to your self-talk. You can transform a fixed mind-set into a growth mind-set with a turn of phrase. For example:

A fixed mind-set says, "I'm not very good at handling conflict."
A growth mind-set says, "I haven't been very good at handling conflict *up to this point*."

Adding the simple phrase "up to this point" or "yet" leaves room for the possibility of change.

Fixed mind-set = Less learning
Growth mind-set = Lifelong learning

Forgive Yourself

You might have turned to this book because you used to have self-confidence, but now it's gone. Maybe you suffered a big setback or failed spectacularly at something that was really important to you, and it's changed your whole sense of self-worth and zapped your willingness to try.

Or maybe not—maybe a lack of self-confidence has plagued you your whole life, and you just don't see yourself as likely to succeed. No matter where you're starting your self-confidence journey, you're going to mess up and you're going to be rejected along the way. We all are! Confidence requires action, and inevitably, some of your actions are going to flop. What you need to do then is forgive yourself.

GUILT VERSUS SHAME

The first step toward learning to forgive yourself is understanding the difference between guilt and shame. Guilt can be a useful emotion when you've done something that hurt someone else. You can look at what you did and say, "This doesn't match up with who I want to be." You can apologize, make it right, and act differently in the future.

Shame stems from a different kind of self-talk. Whereas guilt comes with a growth mind-set ("I did something bad, but I can do better"), shame is an emotional manifestation of a fixed mind-set. Shame says, "This is who I am."

Guilt still feels awful, but it usually comes with acceptance: You know you messed up, and you're going to own it and try to change. Shame, on the other hand, usually leads to resistance. You might lie, run away, blame someone, have an outburst, or otherwise try to get away from facing the situation. Because shame ties up our actions with our self-worth, we fear that when someone sees our shame, they'll know we're broken, inadequate, or "bad."

Everyone feels shame. Many of us have voices in our minds that shame us by echoing messages we heard as kids, and we don't even realize that no one is keeping those messages playing except us. It's time to let go of that self-talk and realize that if you're flawed, struggling, or hurting, you're just part of the human club. Nothing about your appearance, your parenting, your career success, or anything else could cost you your membership and make you unworthy of love.

Forgiving yourself for your flaws isn't just a one-time thing. It's something you have to practice time and time again, because mistakes *will* happen!

Even when you plan carefully, the outside world can throw curveballs your way. It's only natural that sometimes you'll goof. We often believe we have more control over our lives than we truly do; in reality, a change in the weather, a mood swing, or someone's rude comment can throw us off our game. If you're someone who tends to shy away from taking action because you're afraid of messing up, I'll give you some tools to address perfectionism in chapters 5 and 6.

Accepting the fact that you'll make mistakes doesn't mean you stop holding yourself accountable. Instead, it clears up your mind to take meaningful action. If you hurt someone with your mistake, that means apologizing and making amends. If you didn't, it means examining what efforts you made that didn't quite work and seeking feedback on how to do better next time. When you're not spending days obsessing over what you did wrong, you're also more likely to find creative or innovative solutions to a problem. But most importantly, you'll feel more peace.

Practice Self-Compassion

Aikira couldn't get her six-month-old to sleep through the night, and during the day, the baby was so fussy it was hard to go out in public. Although she was exhausted, she forced herself to go to the Parents as Teachers drop-in center one morning. She knew that socialization was important, even for infants, and her husband told her she'd feel better if she got out of the house more. Once there, she tried to mingle with the other parents. She overheard them talking about what parenting books they'd been reading and the latest milestones their babies had achieved. Aikira went home feeling worse than before. She could barely get the laundry done, much less read the latest parenting books. When her husband got home that evening, she fell into a heap, crying, "I'm just a terrible mother."

What do you think Aikira needs?

A   A good night's sleep.
B   To read up on child development.
C   A big dose of self-compassion.

If you answered *A* and *C*, you're right. In this section, you'll learn how self-compassion can step in at your darkest moments, giving you a powerful tool to alleviate painful emotions and situations.

THREE COMPONENTS OF SELF-COMPASSION

Kristin Neff, PhD, one of the pioneers in the field of self-compassion research, has found that there are three important components to self-compassion. The first is mindfulness: simply being aware that you're hurting and in need of attention. The second is kindness: providing yourself the same comfort and encouragement that you would a good friend or a small child. And finally, self-compassion involves a realization that you're not alone; many other people have had similar experiences. This isn't to minimize your personal situation but to let you know that hard times are part of the human condition.

Aikira, the mother of the six-month-old, was so consumed with worry and self-doubt that she hadn't stopped to realize what tremendous pressure she had put on herself. The first step toward more self-compassion would be to take a mindful pause and say to herself, "This is really hard. I haven't had good sleep for months. No one can function well without sleep." When she has thoughts such as, "Why can't my child sleep through the night?" or even, "I hate being a mother," she can notice them without judgment. Next, she can offer herself words of comfort: "It's okay. Being a parent is hard. I'm here for you." It might seem weird to talk to yourself like this, but once you see how helpful it is, you'll be hooked.

Neff has found that a key tenet of compassionate self-talk is tone of voice: Think warm, friendly, and supportive. In addition, making skin contact with yourself, such as putting your hand on your heart or on your forearm, fosters feelings of safety. This physical expression of kindness lets your body know you're on board and ready to help, activating the "tend-and-befriend" response. Finally, Aikira could remind herself that she's not alone. Although those parents at the drop-in center seemed like they had it all together, they likely had their own struggles. Once Aikira learns to accept her painful feelings and give herself the comfort she needs, she'll be able to relax with her child more. It won't magically make her child sleep through the night, but she'll be able to cope more effectively.

BARRIERS TO SELF-COMPASSION

Some people are hesitant to try self-compassion practices, imagining something along the lines of, "If I'm nice to myself, won't I just lie around all day eating chips and watching TV?"

What about you? Check any of the following barriers that might be keeping you from practicing self-compassion:

- ☐ I won't be motivated.
- ☐ I won't get things accomplished.
- ☐ I don't deserve self-compassion.
- ☐ I'll become weak or soft.
- ☐ It feels too indulgent.
- ☐ It might lead to self-pity.

These are not unreasonable fears, as we live in a culture that uses criticism as motivation. To some extent, it works. Think about it: If you have a baseball coach who yells at you, it will probably motivate you in the short term, as you'll want to avoid the yelling and the humiliation. But over time, this can lead to problems. Too much criticism can leave players feeling demoralized, and some will develop performance anxiety.

Hopefully, you've had a coach or a mentor in your life who has done the opposite. Instead of yelling at you when you make a mistake, they say, "Good try. You messed up, but here's what we can do to make it better." The coach doesn't gloss over your weaknesses, but addresses them while avoiding attacking you personally. Kindness and encouragement can get you moving, too.

A growing body of research shows that self-compassion:

Increases productivity. People who use an encouraging self-coaching style find they actually accomplish more.

Decreases procrastination. Self-compassion interrupts the loop between negative self-talk and procrastination, making it more likely you'll stop hesitating and simply jump in to complete those projects you've been avoiding.

Increases creativity. Extending yourself some TLC can lead to accessing higher levels of creativity. You're also more likely to show up and put your work out there.

Here's the key question for you: What kind of coach do you want to be to yourself?

A SELF-COMPASSION BREAK

Try the following exercise:

1. Think of a situation you're struggling with.
2. Assume a posture of self-compassion, such as your hand over your heart.
3. Say to yourself in a kind tone, "This is a moment of suffering," or, "This is really hard right now."
4. Take a few deep breaths and let the words sink in deeply.
5. Say to yourself, "Suffering is a part of life. Other people feel the same way." Take a few more deep breaths.
6. Finally, say to yourself, "May I be kind to myself in this moment and give myself the kindness I need." Repeat these words to yourself as many times as it takes for them to really sink in.

It's all right if you felt a little hokey trying that exercise. In the Resources section (page 153), I list places you can find a variety of self-compassion exercises so you can find ones that feel just right.

Love Yourself

You wouldn't think it would be so hard to love ourselves—flaws and blemishes and all—but somehow, unconditional acceptance eludes us. And yet, to pursue our goals and live a confident life, we need self-love.

It's important to realize that self-love is a process, and we need to start where we are. Not all of us are going to love ourselves with abandon right off the bat, and that's okay.

LOVE IS OUR BIRTHRIGHT

One thing that's helped me and many of my clients is thinking about how we all come into the world the same: helpless, with arms outstretched, *expecting* to be held, fed, and loved. Ideally, a baby is immediately embraced and hears its parents' delight as they say, "Welcome to the world, baby. We're glad you're here." With any luck, our needs are met most of the time. Love is our birthright.

When I worked at a hospital, every time a child was born, a lullaby would play over the loudspeaker. In my current office building, it's a given that when someone is out on parental leave, the parent brings the baby in for a visit at some point. Everyone runs out of their offices to see them, hold the baby, and hear the stories. There's something magical about new life.

What if we could nurture ourselves as we would a newborn baby? What might that feel like? What might that look like? How might our lives be different?

A blogger friend, Kristin Noelle, says it's true that we're born innocent. And, she says, "We are *still* innocent. We make messes of things absolutely, and hurt ourselves and one another in all sorts of ways. But at heart, I believe we're each, given our genetic makeup and life experiences, doing the best we can."

You can take the same approach to learning to love yourself as you're taking to building confidence: If the feelings just aren't there yet, start with actions. This can mean taking care of your body, a topic we'll discuss more in the next chapter. It can also mean making efforts to make your life a little easier or more fun. For example, one simple act of self-love might be picking out the next day's outfit and packing lunches at night to make your morning less stressful. You'll likely find yourself thinking, "Wow, I'm so glad I did that"—a little burst of gratitude that will make you feel more positively toward yourself.

Think about the ways you show love to a significant other or family member. Do you surprise them with flowers, treats, or tickets to see a favorite sports team? Do you make them coffee in the morning or have their favorite meal ready at the end of a long day? Now, think of yourself as your own loved one. What acts of kindness could you do for yourself?

Another strategy is to keep a love list—a list of activities that bring you joy that you can plan to incorporate into your week. These could be things like bubble baths, crossword puzzles, rounds of golf—whatever it is that makes your heart sing. Refer back to it whenever you need a little spiritual boost.

My Love List

THE FEAR FACTOR: PRACTICING ACCEPTANCE

Acceptance can be terrifying when we're used to practicing denial. All of us have had moments when we'd rather run from what's happening than face it. Sometimes we tell ourselves that if we just pretend things are all right, our problems will go away. That's easier than coming to grips with whatever truth scares us, whether it's that we've gained some weight, stayed too long in an unhappy relationship, or fallen on hard times.

But just because you accept something doesn't mean you are surrendering to it, letting it become a permanent part of your life. The sooner you face the monster in the closet, the sooner you'll see it's not as ugly as you thought. You are totally capable of living a full and beautiful life, no matter what lies behind those doors.

Another scary thing about acceptance is that it can mean pushing back against messages from others. Maybe someone in your life tells you that you don't measure up in one way or another, and it takes a lot of courage to push back and say, "Actually, I'm happy with who I am." But you have that courage inside you, and when you let your light shine, you'll be doing a service to yourself and many others.

Take a moment to think about your own fear or trepidation around acceptance. What's stopping you from accepting yourself and your life?

It's okay to be afraid or to worry that you just can't accept yourself. Start with baby steps, and you'll find it becomes more natural over time.

Chapter Takeaways

Self-acceptance is one of the most rewarding principles you can adopt in your life, and it will serve as a foundation for the rest of the confidence skills you'll learn from this book. In the next chapter, I'll show you how to use breathing, posture, and other tools to calm your anxiety and feel more self-assured in any situation.

ACTION ITEMS

Here are some specific actions you can take to implement the lessons and ideas you learned in this chapter:

1. Give yourself some credit: Write down or tell someone three things you did today that went well.
2. The next time you get a compliment, say "thank you" and leave it at that.
3. Do one thing on your love list (see page 64) this week to lift your spirits.
4. Take the Self-Compassion Test online: http://self-compassion.org/test -how-self-compassionate-you-are.
5. Explore self-compassion meditations on the free Insight Timer app.

CHAPTER 4

CALM YOUR BODY

· · · · · · · ·

"OUR BODIES CHANGE OUR MINDS, AND OUR MINDS CAN CHANGE OUR BEHAVIOR, AND OUR BEHAVIOR CAN CHANGE OUR OUTCOMES."

—AMY CUDDY

Andre was the communications director for a large company, but he lost his job in a corporate reorganization. After many years of feeling very comfortable and confident in his position, he was now relegated to scouring online job boards, submitting applications, and hoping his résumé would interest a hiring manager.

Andre's background and résumé attracted considerable interest, and he was invited to several interviews. But each time, something seemed to go wrong. A couple times Andre stumbled while answering a question. On other occasions, he had the gut feeling the employer was looking for someone younger.

Andre began to doubt himself. There must be something wrong with him to get rejected over and over for jobs for which he was highly qualified. When he asked his friends for help, they didn't seem to think the problem was his answers. Instead, it was how he was presenting himself. One friend suggested he shave his beard so he might look more youthful. Another said he needed to be more *outgoing and friendly. His wife pointed out that when he was nervous, he came across as flat and distant. Each piece of well-meaning advice made Andre question more and more how he came across in the interviews. He realized knowing his stuff wasn't going to be enough to land a job. In order to be perceived as confident, he was going to have to fine-tune the messages he was sending with his body language, vocal inflections, and even his grooming.*

In this chapter, you'll see that to build confidence, you have to ready your body as well as your mind. I'll teach you proven ways to calm your body so you can perform at your peak, even during stressful situations such as a job interview. You'll learn powerful mindfulness, gratitude, and relaxation techniques, in addition to gaining tips for general physical self-care. And finally, I'll lead you through some fascinating ways you can use your body posture to soothe your anxiety and express more confidence.

Revisit Your Goals

Do you relate to Andre's story? Think of a time when your body language may have been giving off a less-than-confident vibe or you felt so nervous that you couldn't perform up to your potential. On the lines below, describe what happened and how it felt.

Mindfulness

I touched on mindfulness in chapter 2 and offered you a brief taste of a mindful breathing exercise. Recall that mindfulness is intentionally paying attention to the present moment with an attitude of openness, nonjudgment, and curiosity. It's a way of inclining the mind in a useful direction. You've heard the phrase, "You are what you eat." The same can be said for our minds: We are what we pay attention to. By directing your attention in a certain way, mindfulness will help you develop greater calm at your core, making it more likely you'll tackle even your toughest challenges. A strong mindfulness muscle, built through regular practice, is an important tool to have in your self-confidence tool kit.

Before we move on, I want to dispel a few myths about mindfulness that may get in the way of your approaching this section with an open mind.

MINDFULNESS MYTHS

- You do not have to believe anything in particular to practice mindfulness. Although many religions have contemplative practices (e.g., meditation, centering prayers), the versions you'll learn here are secular.
- Mindfulness is not something exotic, mysterious, or reserved for a special few. You don't have to sit cross-legged, and you don't have to burn incense (but you can if you want to).
- Mindfulness may or may not involve formal meditation. Some people develop a regular meditation practice once they get a taste of mindfulness, but this is not necessary.
- Mindfulness is not a cure-all. As mindfulness has entered the mainstream culture, the implication has been that it's so powerful it can cure everything from depression to chronic pain. While it can help with many conditions, it's generally not a stand-alone treatment. If you suffer from clinical depression or an anxiety disorder, or have a history of trauma, please work with a mental health professional.

Have you tried mindfulness before?

☐ Yes
☐ No

What has been your experience?

☐ Positive
☐ Negative
☐ Neutral

Check any of the mindfulness myths that you've ever believed:

☐ Mindfulness involves religion.
☐ Mindfulness is mysterious.
☐ You have to meditate to practice mindfulness.
☐ Mindfulness will cure all your problems.

MINDFULNESS BASICS

The steps of most mindfulness practices share common instructions:

Bring your attention to the present moment. To facilitate this, you'll select an object of attention. It can be the breath, but it could be the sounds around you, sensations in a part of your body (for example, the hands), or the experience of the whole body.

Observe what's happening in that moment. If you're focusing on the breath, notice where you feel the breath most strongly—at the nostrils, perhaps the chest, or maybe the abdomen. If you'd like, you can silently say, "In," on the inhale and, "Out," on the exhale. This is a soft mental note to help you stay focused. If you're focusing on your hands, you can ask, "Do they feel warm? Are they tingling?" By focusing on your present moment experience, you'll be able to disengage more easily from the past, which you can't change, and the future, which is uncertain.

Notice when your attention has strayed. It may be a few seconds or a few minutes into your practice, but you'll wake up and realize that you've been lost in a long story (what your boss said to you yesterday) or a short complaint (your leg is falling asleep). No problem! It doesn't mean you've done anything wrong. Meditation expert Sharon Salzberg calls this "the magic moment," and believes it to be a crucial aspect of the practice. The point when you notice your mind has wandered is the moment when you have a chance to do it differently. Instead of scolding yourself by thinking, "I am so bad at this," be gentle with yourself and simply start again, refocusing on your object of attention.

That's it. The three basic instructions are simple, although you'll find they're not always easy. Practice helps a lot, and so do the following tips.

MINDFULNESS TIPS

If you're a beginner, here are some practical ways to work mindfulness practices into your daily life. Set a goal to spend just a few minutes being mindful each day. If you want to devote more time to your practice, you can refer to the Resources section (page 153) for books, apps, and podcasts that can help.

Find your style. If you sit at your desk all day, practicing mindfulness on a chair or cushion at home may not be what you need. A walking mindfulness practice may suit you better.

Be flexible. Some people suffer from chronic pain or other health conditions, and prolonged sitting is difficult. Magazine covers show young bodies sitting in the lotus position, but you can practice while sitting, lying down, walking, or standing. Listen to your body, and practice in whatever pose works for you.

Keep your expectations realistic. Remember that mindfulness isn't going to solve all your problems and make your life constantly peaceful.

ONE-MINUTE MINDFULNESS

Here are a few exercises you can try that will take no longer than a minute.

1. Notice that you're safe right now. Are you breathing? Check. Jon Kabat-Zinn reminds us, "If you're breathing, there's more right with you than wrong with you."
2. Take a deep breath, imagining you're breathing in white light as you inhale and breathing out dark clouds as you exhale. Repeat.
3. Pet your cat or dog and immerse yourself in the sensations of your hand touching its fur. Allow your pet's unconditional loving gaze to seep deep inside you.
4. Do this "5-4-3-2-1" exercise that engages all your senses: Take note of five things you can see, four things you can hear, three things you can touch, two things you can smell, and one thing you can taste.
5. Pretend you have to write a letter to a friend describing this moment with as much evocative detail as possible. What do you notice around you? How would you set the scene?
6. Focus for a moment on each part of your body from toes to head, thinking to yourself with each breath, "Let my feet be at ease … Let my calves be at ease … Let my knees be at ease," and so forth.
7. Take a minute during a meal to set distractions aside and focus on the experience of eating. Taking slow bites, notice the aromas and flavors of the dish and the gratitude you feel for the meal.
8. Visualize a stream flowing past you. Each time a thought pops into your head, imagine the thought as a leaf on the stream, slowly passing by and out of view.
9. Think about your hands. What have your hands done for you today? Notice any worries or judgments about each hand. What sensations do you feel in your hands right now? Let your thoughts come and go.
10. Pick an object in your surroundings and pretend you've never seen it before. With openness and curiosity, notice its color, texture, shape, and shadow.

One thing I hope you'll discover: Although you may not find any one mindfulness session particularly impressive, over time, you'll notice the effects in your life. For example, you'll instinctively pause before you hit Send on that critical email, or you'll more quickly refocus when you're being a jerk to yourself. Mindfulness will pave the way to a more positive and confident you.

Relaxation

Stress can make you feel out of control, which undermines self-confidence. When you feel out of your depth or are facing a challenge that matters a lot to you, physical symptoms of anxiety are almost sure to follow. A racing heart and sweaty palms can draw your attention away from the moment, but with some practice, you can learn to soothe yourself through relaxation techniques.

By relaxing, you not only train the body to react differently to events going on around you; you also change the way you think about situations or tasks that used to fill you with dread. As you face these situations and cope better using these relaxation techniques, your fear will lessen and your self-confidence will improve.

DIAPHRAGMATIC BREATHING

In mindfulness practice, we use the breath as an anchor, but we're not trying to manipulate it in any way. We're simply noticing and experiencing the sensations of the breath. There are also formal breathing techniques that can help you focus and calm your nerves, preparing you for whatever confidence challenge you're about to face.

The breathing technique described below is often called *diaphragmatic breathing*, named for the large, umbrella-shaped muscle that separates the chest cavity from the abdominal cavity.

There are four main points to know about diaphragmatic breathing:

1. Inhale and exhale through your nose. Breathing through your mouth increases the possibility of hyperventilating.
2. As you inhale, your abdomen should extend outward. You can think of this as making room for the air you're taking in. As you exhale, your abdomen flattens as you push the air out.
3. Concentrate on slowing down your breathing to approximately 8 to 10 breaths per minute. This is just a general guideline; you don't have to count each time.
4. Make the exhale longer than the inhale. Really work at pushing all the air out of your lungs. For example, if you inhale to the count of four, exhale to the count of six.

One of the easiest ways to learn this form of breathing is to lie on the floor or sit in a chair, with one hand on your abdomen right about where your navel is. Feel your hand rise and fall as you inhale and exhale, following the points above. Practice this twice a day, 5 minutes each time. By deliberately choosing to breathe in a more calming manner, you give yourself the opportunity to think more clearly about your reactions to events, rather than simply responding in a knee-jerk fashion.

Keep track of your practice with the Relaxation Practice Log on the following page.

Use this form to track your breathing and progressive muscle relaxation exercises. Note the date and time, the type of exercise you practiced, and your beginning and ending tension level, with 0 being very relaxed and 10 being very tense.

Date/Time	Type of Exercise	Beginning Tension Level (0-10)	Ending Tension Level (0-10)

PROGRESSIVE MUSCLE RELAXATION

The goal of progressive muscle relaxation is to recognize the difference between how your muscles feel when they're tense and how they feel when relaxed. With practice, you'll begin to quickly scan your body for muscle tension and be able to relax trouble spots on command.

These are the instructions:

1. Find a comfortable, quiet place to sit or lie down.
2. Take a deep breath from your diaphragm (your belly).
3. Tense each muscle group following the list below. Notice what the tension feels like. Hold the tension for 5 to 10 seconds.
4. Release the tension. Focus on how relaxed the muscle feels.
5. Take another deep breath.
6. Repeat the procedure with each muscle group.

Below are the major areas of the body. If you experience pain in any of the areas, stop immediately and omit them in the future.

- Right foot, then left foot
- Right calf, then left calf
- Right thigh, then left thigh
- Hips and buttocks
- Stomach
- Chest
- Back
- Right arm and hand, then left arm and hand
- Neck and shoulders
- Face

It should take approximately 15 to 20 minutes to go through the entire process. Remember, the goal is to really notice the difference between tension and relaxation.

Once you gain some comfort with progressive muscle relaxation, you can omit the tensing part, and instead focus only on relaxing each area of the body in turn. Silently tell yourself to relax each muscle and allow the tension to slip effortlessly away. You can intensify the relaxation by imagining the muscle being heavy and warm. This will shorten the time the process takes and allow you to reach a state of relaxation more quickly.

Keep track of your practice on the same Relaxation Practice Log that you used for your diaphragmatic breathing exercises.

Gratitude

Gratitude can be one of the most calming practices you can adopt, particularly when you think you don't have much to be thankful for. As you learned in chapter 3, our minds are wired to zoom in on negative events, blurring out the bounty of blessings surrounding them. If you're holding this book, you likely also have access to food, shelter, sanitation, and safety. How lucky is that? Our fears tend to loom large, but practicing gratitude can help us zoom out and see them in the context of everything that's going right.

GRATITUDE FOR THE POSITIVE

Low self-confidence often goes hand in hand with a mentality of scarcity. We think we don't have enough beauty, enough brains, enough discipline, or enough moxie to be where we want to be. But in reality, most of us are surrounded by abundance. Try this: When you find yourself focusing on an area where you think you're lacking, replace it with thoughts about what you do have.

Here's an example:

Scarcity thought: I don't make as much money as the other people in my social circle.
Abundance thoughts: I have a job. I put food on the table. I have a home. I buy clothes for my kids. I have a comfortable bed. I have a phone and a TV. I have the means to visit out-of-state relatives every year. (And so on.)

Now you try:

Scarcity thought:

_____

_____

Abundance thoughts:

_____

_____

_____

Research shows practicing gratitude decreases rumination, increases energy, and contributes to overall happiness. It also improves sleep; many people find it useful to write in a gratitude journal before bed. You can also trade the old trick of counting sheep for counting blessings, which replaces the anxious thoughts that tend to creep in at night with thoughts of gratitude for the health, love, safety, fun, and meaning in your life.

GRATITUDE AFTER TRAUMA

We've all had deeply painful experiences we wish we could go back in time and erase: the death of a loved one, a terrible injury, a failed marriage. Such experiences can shift our life paths and fundamentally change who we are. These are the dark parts of life that can keep us trudging along old roads of pain, fear, and self-doubt.

But it's possible to modify your mind-set to focus on what happened in the *aftermath* of the terrible event. Our greatest challenges often show us strength we never knew we had. We gain perspective and start treating life as precious and fleeting. We're gentler and kinder to others. Our skin gets thicker. We learn who really cares for us and what we're truly made of. We see flaws in the path we had been headed down before we were forced onto a new one.

Research on post-traumatic growth shows that practicing gratitude for those changes can make us more resilient, less fearful, less vengeful, and less stuck in the past. Take note: No one expects you to feel grateful for the negative event itself. While you may eventually view some painful life experiences as blessings in disguise, other things will always be tragedies. But by recognizing the wonderful things in your life that bloomed from those dark days, you're more likely to be able to face the unknown future with openness and bravery.

GRATITUDE FOR OTHERS

Expressing your gratitude for the people in your life is one of the healthiest gratitude practices of all. Not only do you get all the aforementioned benefits of feeling grateful, but you also get to make others feel appreciated—which bolsters your confidence by making you feel like a good person and strengthens your social bonds, lowering your risk of anxiety and depression.

Try incorporating the power of saying "thanks" into your daily life. Give yourself extra points when you:

- ☐ Make your thank-you specific, e.g.: "I really appreciate the work you did on that report, Tina. The extra effort you put into the graphs really made it pop."
- ☐ Thank someone who might not always receive appreciation, such as a janitor or bus driver.
- ☐ Mail an old-school, handwritten thank-you note to someone who has really done a lot for you, perhaps with flowers or another gift.
- ☐ Thank someone who would otherwise have no idea the impact they made on your life. This could be a teacher you had decades ago who shaped your career aspirations or a journalist you've never met whose stories keep you informed about your neighborhood.
- ☐ If you're thanking someone you're close with, do it with a consenual hug or another display of affection. Studies show that holding someone's hand can diminish the experience of physical pain. Just ask first!

Body Language

Remember Andre, our friend from the beginning of this chapter who was struggling with job interviews? He knew his résumé was getting him a second look,
but something about how he was coming off in person was leaving potential employers less than impressed. The more he worried about that, the less
he could focus on selling himself as a candidate. Luckily, science is on Andre's
side—and yours.

When you practice using posture and nonverbal communication to your
advantage, not only will you appear more confident to others, but you'll feel more
confident, too. That's because the way you stand, sit, and move sends signals to
your brain about whether there's a threat in your environment. When you learn to
calm your mind, you can free yourself up to concentrate on what really matters,
like wowing an interviewer.

NONVERBAL COMMUNICATION

If you struggle with confidence, sometimes your body can feel traitorous. You're
convinced everyone can see how nervous you are; your fears and flaws are radi-
ating through every pore. It's true that nonverbal communication makes a strong
impression: Studies show eye contact, facial expressions, gestures, and posture
send more memorable messages than words. But the good news is that you have
a lot of control over the signals you're sending, and projecting confidence is not
as difficult as you might think.

The two key concepts to remember are *openness* and *warmth*. If you can
keep those traits in mind, your authentic and best self will shine through, allowing you to be seen, heard, and truly understood by others.

Openness: When you find a situation threatening, your body's instinct is to
retreat into itself. Without realizing it, you might find yourself slouching,
folding your arms across your chest, or placing a hand on your neck. Those
movements keep your body in fight-or-flight mode, paralyzing you with

anxiety. Remind yourself instead to take up space. Follow your grandmother's advice: Sit up straight, uncross your arms and legs, and try not to fidget. Take up time, too, breathing deeply and speaking without rushing.

Warmth: Research shows people feel instantly connected with someone who acts warm and friendly. Once that person is in their good graces, they don't pay much mind to conversational stumbles, a cracking voice, or a trembling hand. So when you feel intimidated, remember that you already know how to be kind. Smile, ask questions, include people, and look them in the eye. It makes a world of difference.

If you'd like, you can ask a trusted friend or family member to tip you off to body language cues you don't know you're sending. Nervous habits, like peeling the label off a beer bottle at happy hour, can sometimes become invisible to us. These small habits may seem unimportant, but keep in mind that all of this work is in the service of getting your values and strengths to shine through.

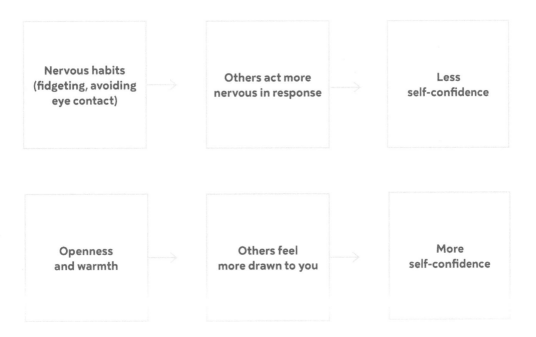

Nervous habits (fidgeting, avoiding eye contact) → Others act more nervous in response → Less self-confidence

Openness and warmth → Others feel more drawn to you → More self-confidence

If you've seen psychologist Amy Cuddy's viral 2012 TED Talk, "Your Body Language May Shape Who You Are," you know there's even more you can do to use your body to psych up your mind. Cuddy popularized the idea of "power posing," or holding yourself in an expansive posture for a couple minutes before you walk into a confidence challenge. It sounds silly, but it works: The pose shifts your hormonal balance, making you feel more powerful and more likely to take risks.

Now, Cuddy doesn't recommend standing like Wonder Woman at the front of a crowded boardroom. But if you can find a bathroom stall or another private place to "power pose" just before a big interview, presentation, or date, you'll reap physiological rewards. Here are two poses you can try:

Wonder Woman: Stand with your feet shoulder-width apart, chest puffed out and hands on your hips, like a superhero.

Starfish: This is the ecstatic pose you see when people cross the finish line of a race. With your feet shoulder-width apart, hold your arms in a *V* over your head, making yourself as big as you can.

Maintain Your Physical Health

If you find yourself having trouble staying calm under pressure, you might be surprised how much of a difference it makes to treat your body well. Sometimes that means a big mind-set shift is in order, because to give your body what it needs, you have to put yourself first. Too often we don't take time to exercise or enjoy something relaxing because we're too busy putting other people's needs ahead of our own. When I fall into that trap, I recall the preflight instructions on airlines: Put your own oxygen mask on first.

SLEEP

Many of us are chronically sleep-deprived. We stay up late to finish that report, do another load of laundry, or zone out behind our screens.

For people prone to self-doubt, adequate sleep is crucial. It can mean the difference between thinking about an issue realistically and becoming needlessly upset over something that's not important.

How much sleep is enough? Although many people require approximately seven to eight hours each night, individual needs vary. The general rule of thumb is if you're sleepy during the day, you probably need more sleep. Sticking to a regular bedtime and wake-up time also makes a big difference.

Many sleep experts also recommend a 20- to 30-minute nap during the afternoon, citing improved concentration and functioning. Unfortunately, corporate America doesn't generally allow for this. But if you work at home and can take a quick catnap, it's definitely worth trying.

Before you fall asleep, take a few moments to dwell on a sense of peacefulness, noting that nothing is wrong or missing. Sure, maybe the day had its challenges, but you're safe now, and all your basic needs are met. Bring to mind the people you care about, and those who care about you, as you gently allow yourself to let go of the day.

EXERCISE

Have you ever felt stuck on a problem—be it a work project or a battle of wills with a toddler—and then gone for a walk or a run, only to return with a clear mind, knowing just what to do?

That's the power of exercise. It's definitely more than getting in shape. It's an integral part of reducing tension and worry, managing negative moods, and as noted above, problem solving. Coping with stress by engaging the body is great because you bypass a lot of unhelpful mental chatter. The key is finding a form of activity you enjoy that doesn't feel boring or like a chore you have to do because "it's good for you."

For aerobic exercise, try swimming, running, or walking. Consider yoga or tai chi for exercise that taps strongly into the mind–body connection. If you enjoy team sports, check around for a recreational league. And don't forget about activities you enjoyed as a child that you can still do now: riding a bike, dancing, or chasing after your dog in the backyard.

HEALTHFUL EATING

I wish I could tell you there's a perfect confidence diet, but no such luck. Everyone has to figure out for themselves what foods make them feel their best. Of course, we all benefit from plenty of healthy, nutrient-dense food, but that doesn't mean you can't enjoy your favorite treats on occasion. Eating should be enjoyable; if you find that your relationship with food has become obsessive or stressful, please consider talking to your doctor. There are additional resources related to disordered eating in the back of this book (see page 153).

At the risk of sounding preachy, keep in mind that some foods and substances can be confidence killers if overdone. For example, while coffee in moderation can improve focus, too much can lead to jitters. In addition to coffee, watch your intake of alcohol. Many people with low self-confidence, particularly in social situations, use alcohol to cope. Sadly, the things that people do to cope with social anxiety, such as having a drink or two *before* the party, will only maintain fear over the long run.

THE FEAR FACTOR: CALMING YOUR BODY

Some of what I've discussed in this chapter might not sound like fun to you. For instance, some people who have tried breathing exercises or mindfulness don't find them soothing at all at first. "What's so calming about being alone with my racing thoughts?" you might think. Or maybe sitting there with your eyes closed just makes you feel a little silly.

If sitting still doesn't come naturally to you, and you've never had any success clearing your mind, you are 100 percent normal. The goal here is not to become a Zen master, unless you really want to! Instead, you're simply trying to make your body a little bit more of an ally as you pursue your goals.

The suggestions in this chapter also include some lifestyle changes that might seem overwhelming. Please don't worry that you'll never attain self-assurance until you're a marathon-running, caffeine-eschewing, vegan yogi who has no trouble sleeping through the night. You don't have to be in perfect health to be confident—in fact, you don't have to be a perfect anything to be confident! When it comes to being kind to your body, small changes can make a world of difference.

Take a moment to note any fears or trepidation that arose as you read this chapter, and then note three baby steps you can take to overcome those fears.

Chapter Takeaways

In this chapter, you learned how observing the present moment can stop your mind from time traveling to the past and future. You saw how your breathing, posture, and other nonverbal cues can trick your body into telling your mind to calm down. Maybe you're even appreciating your mom for her age-old advice to say "thank you" and to get some sleep, because now you know how those habits boost confidence.

Now that you know your body a bit better, it's time to get to know your mind. Let's look at how negative thinking can trap us and keep us from progressing toward our goals and becoming more confident, and how we can overcome it.

ACTION ITEMS

Here are some specific actions you can take to implement the lessons and ideas you learned in this chapter:

1. When you next find yourself with a few minutes of downtime—maybe when you're waiting in line—try one of the one-minute mindfulness exercises (page 72) from this chapter.
2. See if you can incorporate 90 minutes of exercise into your week.
3. Say, "Thank you," to someone you've never thanked before.
4. Watch Amy Cuddy's talk about "power posing" on TED.com.
5. Set a goal to go to bed and wake up at the same time every day this week.

CHAPTER 5

WORK WITH YOUR THOUGHTS

. . . .

*"IT IS THE MARK OF AN EDUCATED MIND TO BE ABLE
TO ENTERTAIN A THOUGHT WITHOUT ACCEPTING IT."*

—ARISTOTLE

There's no way I'll get that promotion.
I'm failing as a parent.
No one would want to go out with me. I'm such a loser.

Does any of this sound familiar? If so, you're not alone. Many people battle negative thinking constantly.

Unfortunately, most of us don't know how to handle negative thinking in a healthy way. We obsess over the reasons we can't do something or aren't good enough, working ourselves into an anxious frenzy that affects our performance. Our preoccupation with the worst-case scenario becomes a self-fulfilling prophecy, lowering our self-confidence and keeping us from doing our best.

This chapter introduces one approach to dealing with negative thoughts and the self-talk that results from those thoughts. You will learn how to identify unhelpful thinking patterns and how to consider other, more adaptive ways of thinking. As you examine and question your negative thoughts, you may find deeper assumptions at their root. I'll talk more about how to address negative core beliefs in chapter 6.

Keep in mind that this chapter is not about going to war with your negative thoughts. It's about recognizing them and considering alternative possibilities, freeing yourself up to take action and build self-confidence.

Revisit Your Goals

Take some time to revisit the goals you set for yourself in chapter 2. Are there any negative thoughts holding you back from pursuing those goals? What are they? If you could rise above them, what kind of difference do you think that would make in your life? Jot down some thoughts below.

The Trap of Negative Thinking

All of us have a near-constant stream of thoughts running through our minds. Much of the time, these thoughts are neutral, and sometimes they're even pleasant. The thoughts we'll be dealing with are what psychologists call *automatic negative thoughts* or *cognitive distortions*. These are thoughts that don't serve you well. They're either blatantly untrue or, at the very least, not helpful.

Negative thoughts themselves aren't the problem—it's the power we give them. You can choose to believe your negative thoughts, treating them as unassailable facts and proceeding through life trapped in their iron grip. Or you can choose to perceive a negative thought the same way you view the millions of fleeting sensations, snap judgments, and other cognitions that zip through your mind every day. They're information, sure, but they're not absolute truth.

To help you recognize and deconstruct your negative thoughts, let's learn about the different flavors these thoughts come in. We'll focus on the story of Sasha, a 40-year-old woman who dreams of going back to school to earn her bachelor's degree but just can't shake her nagging doubts.

MAKING ASSUMPTIONS

"If I go back to school, all the 18-year-olds in my classes will judge me and pity me for being there. Plus, I haven't been in school for decades. I'm so out of practice that I'll fail all my classes."

When Sasha thinks about college, she immediately jumps to conclusions. She can see into the future, and it's not pretty. But what evidence does she really have to believe this unfortunate vision of her collegiate career? When you make assumptions, you're usually filling the void of the unknown by imagining an undesirable outcome. In reality, a number of good things are also possible.

"SHOULDING"

"A person my age should be making twice as much money as I am now. I need to get my act together."

Sasha's stress about her education level sometimes bubbles up into thoughts about where she "should" be in life or what she "needs" or "ought" to do. This type of thinking might almost sound positive: Hey, she's motivating herself to pursue a goal, right? But what she's really doing here is setting inflexible standards for herself that she's already failed to meet. Her "shoulding" isn't rooted in self-compassion or her own values; the goalpost is arbitrary.

When Sasha really thinks about what matters to her, her salary is nowhere near the top of the list. She wants an education to better herself and pursue a more meaningful career. Her "shoulds" come from internalizing others' expectations and comparing herself to her neighbor down the street, and listening to those thoughts has only convinced her she'll never measure up. That perfectionism is bound to shake her self-confidence and make it harder to move toward her goals.

BLACK-AND-WHITE/ALL-OR-NOTHING THINKING

"If I don't graduate with honors at the end of all this, it won't have been worth the struggle. I'll be a failure."

Here, Sasha has decided that she's either an A+ or an F. There is no in between. This kind of perfectionism sets her up to view herself as a failure no matter what. But the truth is there's a lot of beauty between these two poles, where she'll most likely end up: the concepts she'll conquer, the skills she'll gain, the pride she'll feel knowing she went for her goal. She will make mistakes, but they won't reduce her to a zero. Learning to appreciate her accomplishments without letting her false steps overshadow them will allow her to keep moving forward.

CATASTROPHIZING

"If I enroll in college full-time, I'm just going to flunk out my first semester, and I won't be able to come back to this job. Then I'll run out of money. I'll have to move in with my mother, and I'll be so ashamed I'll just want to lie down and die."

IDENTIFY AND RECORD NEGATIVE THOUGHTS

Just as tracking your spending helps you stick to a budget, writing down your negative thoughts will help you take inventory of what's running through your mind and why. Try keeping a log of your automatic negative thoughts for a few days. This works best if you carry a small notebook with you, so you can capture the thought when it's fresh in your mind.

Record the uncensored version of what's going on in your mind. What are you telling yourself? What do you fear will happen? If you're having trouble putting it into words, write anyway: "I'm not sure what I'm thinking, but I wonder if it has something to do with _____?" Generate several possibilities.

You won't have to write out your thoughts forever. But in the beginning, most people find it helpful. Sometimes, as soon as you write down a thought, you're able to catch the error in your logic. ("Wait, why am I assuming my boss will be angry if I ask for guidance on this project? Maybe she'll be glad to help.") Other times, you might need to examine the thought more to evaluate whether it's realistic and what you can do about it. Or the thought might be linked to a faulty core belief, such as, "A good employee never asks for help." I'll help you learn to dig deeper into your thoughts and beliefs in this chapter and the next.

Sasha's worrying mind has leapt from merely making assumptions to imagining the worst-case scenario, a failure so devastating she could never recover. The chances that bright and driven Sasha will fail out of school, fail to find work, and wind up back at her mother's house are so miniscule as to be laughable. But when she buys into what her mind is telling her, she sometimes loses sight of reality.

"Whenever I even think about walking into a college classroom, I feel embarrassed, stupid, and panicked. That just goes to show this is a bad idea and I could never hack it."

It's all too easy for Sasha to let her feelings write the story of what her college experience would be like. If she feels stupid, that must mean she is stupid. But feelings aren't facts.

If you want to prove it to yourself, think about the last time you dealt with a week of rainy weather. After a day or two, you probably felt a little glum, and maybe your inner monologue started to sound like it was written by Eeyore, the sad-sack donkey from *Winnie-the-Pooh*: "Oh, why bother? Nothing ever goes right for me." But nothing about your life had actually changed. You were just buying into your feelings, which can shift with your hormones, your diet, and even the weather.

"FEAR IS FAMILIARITY'S IMPOSTER. IT PASSES OFF WHAT YOU DREAD FOR WHAT YOU KNOW. OFFERS THE WORST IN PLACE OF THE AMBIGUOUS. SERVES UP ANXIETY IN THE ABSENCE OF COMFORT. SUBSTITUTES ASSUMPTION FOR REASON. UNDER THE WARPED LOGIC OF FEAR, ANYTHING IS BETTER THAN THE UNCERTAIN."

—ISAAC LIDSKY

Our feelings love to spin narratives about whether we'll succeed and whether others like us. But often, these stories are wildly off the mark.

Now that you know some of the key types of automatic negative thoughts, see if you can recognize them in your own thinking. Pick one of your goals from your list in chapter 2. Think about the process of chasing that goal, and using the space below, list any negative thoughts and predictions that come to mind.

Next, examine each thought and see if it fits into one or more of the cognitive distortion categories discussed in this chapter.

Negative Thoughts	Cognitive Distortions

6 Steps to Break Negative Thinking Patterns

Once you've started noticing your negative thoughts, you're well on your way to breaking free of them. Don't get frustrated if you find it challenging at first. As you know, our minds are wired to focus on the negative. Just as memories are tagged by smell and taste, they're also tagged by feeling, meaning that once you're in a bad mood, it's easy to get caught in a negative thought spiral. You might feel a little like Michael Corleone in *The Godfather Part III*: "Just when I thought I was out, they pull me back in!" But the techniques in this section will help you train your brain to draw itself out of the muck.

IDENTIFY THINKING ERRORS

Automatic negative thoughts can be like a loud air conditioner or a noisy street. You get so used to hearing them drone on, day in and day out, that at some point you don't even realize they're there. That's why it's useful to get in the habit of writing them down. Suddenly, the ceaseless background noise saying, "Am I enough? Am I doing this right? Will they like me?" comes into the foreground, making it easier to address.

It would be nice if a thinking error would sound an alert, saying, "Hey, don't believe me. I'm an automatic negative thought." But too often, we're not initially aware that we're in distorted-thinking territory. We might not even "hear" the thought in distinct, easy-to-express words. Pay attention to your feelings. If you notice a change in your mood or an increase in anxiety, ask yourself, "What was I doing just before I felt anxious? What was going on around me?" Take a mindful pause and see what arises, remembering not to judge your thoughts.

When you write down the thoughts, ask yourself, "What evidence is there to support this idea? What evidence is there against it?" See if you can match the thought to one of the cognitive distortions listed above. Use the following chart to identify negative thoughts and examine them. Take your time over the course of a week or so; each time a negative thought arises, jot it down in the chart.

Automatic negative thought	Evidence this is true	Evidence this is false

REFRAME NEGATIVE SELF-TALK

Sometimes, asking whether a negative thought is realistic is enough to dismantle it. That approach works particularly well with thoughts about outcomes: If you're expecting failure, you can usually push yourself to see that success is possible, too. But with other types of thoughts, asking, "Is this true?" is going to leave you spinning your wheels. For instance, if you keep thinking, "I'm ugly," you don't want to spend time looking for objective evidence about whether you're attractive. You'll never find it.

Instead, you want to ask yourself a different question: "Is this thought helpful?" Is it helping you move toward your goals, or is it holding you back? Is it even important or relevant to what you're trying to achieve? Does it sound like something a good coach would say to help motivate you?

If not, try to reframe the thought in a more positive way. Let's say you were taking lessons to learn to swim as an adult. You might think, "I'm so ignorant. I can't believe I'm struggling to learn to do something my six-year-old niece can do!" How does calling yourself dumb make you feel? Is it useful? Not really—if you feel embarrassed for even trying, you're just going to want to quit. Try telling yourself instead, "I'm courageous for taking this step to gain a skill I've always wanted to have."

Reframing works for nerves, too. The next time you're anxious, try telling yourself, "I feel this way because what I'm about to do is important to me. It's great that I'm moving ahead toward my goal." The butterflies in your stomach won't go away, but they'll start to feel a little more like excitement, and you'll remember how prepared and capable you are.

Try reframing some of your own negative thoughts in the space below.

Negative self-talk	What would a friend or wise mentor say?

You've heard the expression, "Don't believe everything you read." Well, it's important not to believe everything you think, either. These techniques can help you defuse from a negative thought, or become less attached to it so you can move forward.

Label your thoughts. Instead of saying, "I'm a loser," say, "I'm having the thought that I'm a loser." Instead of saying, "I'm going to blow this test," say "I'm having the thought that I'm going to blow this test." You can distance the thought even further by saying, "My mind is having the thought that . . . " The difference may seem subtle, but it can help you gain the perspective that you are not your thoughts.

Let them float away. This one involves imagery. You visualize each negative thought as a balloon and imagine it floating up, up, and away. When you have another thought, as you will, you put it on another balloon and watch it float away.

Thank your mind. If you're having anxious thoughts, such as, "I hope this plane doesn't crash . . . I hope the pilot knows what he's doing," say, "Thank you, mind. Thank you for trying to keep me safe. But there's nothing that you really need to do right now. I've got it covered."

Name your stories. Many times, our thoughts are repetitive and involve the same stories. Maybe yours is, "I don't really know what I'm doing." When thoughts come up along that story line, you can say, "Oh, here's my 'I'm Incompetent' story," and just let it go.

Sing your thoughts. Try singing your thoughts to the alphabet song or to "Row, Row, Row Your Boat." Your thoughts will certainly sound absurd this way, which is the whole point.

Now let's put these techniques into practice with an exercise. Think of a negative thought you've had recently, and go through the defusion techniques listed above, one by one. Then use the chart below to rate each technique according to its helpfulness.

Defusion Technique	Not helpful	Somewhat helpful	Very helpful
Label your thoughts			
Let them float away			
Thank your mind			
Name your stories			
Sing your thoughts			

AVOID GENERALIZATIONS

As you get in the habit of noticing your negative thoughts, look for absolute terms, such as *all*, *every*, *none*, *never*, and *always*. Those words usually indicate black-and-white thinking, where you're viewing the world through dark glasses that block out all the good. To switch out your lenses, try to make your self-talk balanced and as specific as possible, as in the examples below. If you're stuck, remind yourself of something you did that went well or an area in which you've made progress.

Generalization: I always screw things up.
Balanced self-talk: Sometimes things don't go as I had planned. Sometimes things go okay. Sometimes things even go better than expected.

Generalization: I'm fat. I'm never going to get in shape.
Balanced self-talk: I weigh 162 pounds, which is less than I did at the beginning of the year. My doctor says my blood pressure is good. Yes, I would benefit from moving more to have more energy, but I've made a good start by adding a 15-minute walk around my neighborhood to my morning routine.

Generalization: I'm always so quiet at parties.
Balanced self-talk: I am often quiet at parties where I don't know many people. Once I get to know someone, I have plenty to say.

You try:

Generalization:

_____

_____

Balanced self-talk:

_____

_____

It's also important to keep a clear, balanced outlook about your future. You might think you know the ending to your story: "Things will never turn out right for me." But the truth is, unless you're psychic, you just can't predict what's going to happen. *Uncertainty* sounds uncomfortable, but it's really another word for *possibility*. The plot twists life has in store can be more thrilling and astonishing than any movie.

Try adding the phrase "I wonder" to the stories you tell yourself about the future: "I wonder how _____ will turn out." If you start to stress about unknowns and what-ifs, tell yourself, "I don't have to know that yet." All you can do is try your best to prepare and feel proud of yourself for doing so.

CALM YOUR INNER CRITIC

Your inner critic is going to be with you your whole life—but that doesn't mean he or she gets to have any power. Here are some ways to push past the nasty words inside your head and keep going.

Give your inner critic a name. "Hey, Negative Nancy, nice to see you again. Why don't you have a seat here and have some tea. Hang out while I do what I need to do." Humor helps!

Remember that your critic has good intentions. For example, maybe your inner critic says, "Don't do that stand-up comedy open mic night. You'll be horrible." The message is meant to save you from embarrassment—but you know better than to let the potential for failure stop you. Don't fight the thoughts, or your inner critic will get louder. Say, "Thanks, mind," and move on.

Remind your inner critic that plenty of times, things turn out just fine. Your inner critic loves to ask, "What if things go wrong?" You can retort, "Well, what if things go right?"

HEALTHY COPING STATEMENTS

Although generalized affirmations, such as, "I'm a winner," don't tend to work to combat negative thinking, there are coping statements you can use to calm yourself down. Like an affirmation, a coping statement is positive. But it's also rooted in what you truly believe, making your mind more likely to buy in.

When you're imagining the worst, try to focus on a coping statement, such as, "Most people will accept it if . . ." ("I stutter during my speech," "my small talk is awkward at the party," or whatever outcome you fear). And then remind yourself, "If not, I can cope"—whether the outcome is disapproval, disappointment, or some other unfavorable result.

Let's look at Mia's example. She had been invited to a pool party and she really wanted to go. She hadn't been out of the house much since her baby was born three months ago, and she wanted to see her friends. The problem was, she "felt fat." She assumed she'd be at her pre-pregnancy weight by now, but she wasn't. How could she possibly be seen in a swimming suit? Her negative thinking was loud and mean: "Everyone will stare at me. They'll think I should've already lost this weight." Mia went through the steps above and made considerable progress in balancing her negative thoughts with more realistic ones. However, when she got stressed thinking about it, all rationality went out the window. She had no confidence in her ability to actually show up—maybe she'd make up an excuse and skip it. So she developed a coping card that she could refer to in the days leading up to the party:

> Most people aren't going to be looking at me; they're going to be talking and having fun. I'm expecting too much of myself. I'm going to go and enjoy myself. Its highly unlikely anyone would really say or think badly of me, but if they do, that's their problem.

How Your Thoughts Impact Your Confidence

Sasha, the aspiring college student from the beginning of this chapter, began to recognize the errors in her thinking. She decided to start the process of applying to a local college. It wasn't easy. Every time she sat down to work on her admissions essay, the gremlins of self-doubt popped into her mind, yelling, "You'll never be able to do this!" Sasha heard the words and said, "Thanks, mind, but I've got this," and carried on writing.

On the day she was finally ready to click the submit button on her online application, Sasha was still anxious. But she was no longer convinced she'd fail. Drawing on her mindfulness skills, Sasha told herself, "We'll see how this goes. It would be wonderful if I got in, but I'm proud of myself just for trying." It felt great to know that she had really "walked her talk": She had always touted the value of education to her children, and she had always wanted to better herself. Now, she was really doing it.

Sasha felt herself growing more self-assured in other areas of her life, too. When she felt incompetent at her job, she recognized the pangs of self-recrimination as the words of her inner critic: just thoughts, not reality. "After all," Sasha thought, "I am still me." Deep down, she knew she had value as a human being, whether or not she ever succeeded in earning a degree. We all have an inner core that doesn't care about our mistakes, our moods, our looks, or our status in society. That part of us always knows our worth. When, like Sasha, we rise above negative and unrealistic thinking, we can live authentically as that core self.

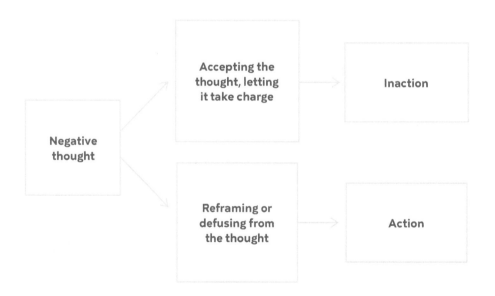

Self-Compassion Revisited

Now that you know how to turn down the volume on your inner critic, remember to add some positivity to your day whenever possible. Here are some strategies to use self-compassion to help you gain the confidence to keep pushing toward your goals.

GIVE YOURSELF A BREAK

Sometimes on your path toward your goals, you're just going to be tapped out. You'll make silly mistakes, struggle to concentrate, or just feel too spent to keep trying. Give yourself permission to have those days. Don't worry; they'll pass. Be kind to yourself the same way you'd be kind to a loved one, and say, "You did a lot today. Sit back, enjoy a drink and a TV show, and try again tomorrow." Everyone needs rest.

What are a few of your favorite ways to recharge after an exhausting day?

RECORD YOUR ACCOMPLISHMENTS

When you're looking up the mountain at how far you still have to go, it's easy to forget how far you've already come. But glancing down the slope you've already climbed is an enormous confidence booster. It's a reminder: "Hey, if I can make it that far, maybe I really can reach the top!" Try recording your accomplishments about once a week in a notebook. Give yourself permission to think small: Maybe you had coffee with someone in another industry to discuss switching careers, or you stood up for yourself when your sister made a disparaging remark about you. Taking those little steps, again and again, is what leads to big change.

When you're feeling overwhelmed by a goal, it helps to remember the adage, "How do you eat an elephant? One bite at a time." Try writing down the steps you'd have to take to be where you want to be. It's okay if some of those steps are just big question marks. You'll fill in those blanks by researching, talking to people, and gaining experience. For now, just look at the first step. *That's all you have to do.*

Say your goal is to train for a marathon. Some mornings you might wake up and think, "I can't do this!" Ask yourself, "What can't I do? Put on my running shoes and go outside? That's all I have to do right now." If you'd started first grade by thinking about how hard your senior year of high school would be, you'd probably be a six-year-old dropout! But by the time you'd finished 11th grade, the 12th grade didn't seem so bad. Have faith that the rungs of the ladder hang together and will get you to the place you're trying to go.

THE FEAR FACTOR:
WORKING WITH YOUR THOUGHTS

Confronting negative thoughts often feels like a Sisyphean task. You keep trying to work with your inner critic, and it just pushes you back down the hill to start over again. That frustration can turn into fear: "What if I'm *always* going to be paralyzed by negative thoughts?"

You might also be afraid that by pushing back against your negative thoughts, you're just kidding yourself. If you stop listening to the voice that says you'll never be good enough, then you'll go out and try something new, and you might fall flat on your face. "See?" you'll think. "I should have known I couldn't do this!"

Write down some of your own fears that arose while you were reading this chapter.

_____

_____

_____

Now, since I'm preaching realistic thinking in this chapter, I'll be honest: Self-doubt will always be a part of your life. (There's a name for the small percentage of people who don't experience any self-doubt: psychopaths.) But that doesn't mean your inner critic will always be in the control tower of your mind. If you keep practicing the skills you learned in this chapter, little by little, you'll learn to keep moving forward despite what Negative Nancy (or Neil) tells you.

And yes, that means sometimes you'll mess up. There's no such thing as progress without some mistakes here and there. Don't let the fear of falling keep you from ever taking your first step.

Chapter Takeaways

Master the art of talking to yourself. Yes, it *sounds* strange, but you know better. Having a healthy dialogue with your negative thoughts helps you poke holes in them, dismiss them when they're not useful, and step over them on your merry way to your goals. In the next chapter, you'll work on some of the stories you tell yourself that are at the root of some of those negative thoughts: the core beliefs that shape your self-image.

ACTION ITEMS

Here are some specific actions you can take to implement the lessons and ideas you learned in this chapter:

1. Some people find it helpful to physically dispose of negative thoughts. Write down a negative thought on a piece of paper, then cut it up and throw it in the trash or carefully burn it.
2. Tell someone close to you that you're trying to reframe your negative thoughts. Ask them to gently let you know when they catch you voicing a self-defeating viewpoint.
3. If you've started to "name your stories" and you're noticing themes around certain repetitive thoughts, write them down. Those themes will help you identify your core beliefs in the next chapter.
4. Reflect on a time when you had a lot of negative predictions about how something would go, and then it wound up going just fine. Hold on to that story the next time your mind is flooding with worries about a future event.
5. Celebrate your victories! If you push past a swarm of negative thoughts to take action toward your goals, give yourself a reward.

CHAPTER SIX

WORK WITH YOUR BELIEFS

. . . .

"THIS IS HOW HUMANS ARE: WE QUESTION ALL OUR BELIEFS, EXCEPT FOR THE ONES THAT WE REALLY BELIEVE IN, AND THOSE WE NEVER THINK TO QUESTION."

—ORSON SCOTT CARD

If you've ever been to therapy, you know that a negative thought rarely stands alone. When you start examining your thinking, you realize it's just a branch of a much more deeply rooted tree. You climb downward and downward, asking yourself, "Why do I think that? Who says? Where is this coming from?" Finally, you arrive at the base of the tree and have your breakthrough, recognizing how a tiny seed planted long ago grew to shape your worldview. The roots of this tree are your negative core beliefs.

For example, when Jasmin's friends talked about their blissful relationships, she found herself becoming more and more agitated. She knew she should feel happy for them, but instead, she just felt alienated. Her boyfriend criticized her

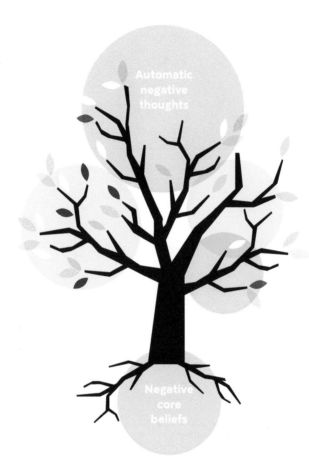

Automatic negative thoughts

Negative core beliefs

constantly and made her feel like her opinions were worthless. Jasmin's friends had told her more than once that she should move on. But she'd always instantly say, "Oh, no, I could never leave him."

One day, her friends pushed back: "Why not?" they said. "What would happen if you did?" Jasmin broke down in tears. She'd never admitted this to anyone, but she really believed that if she broke up with her boyfriend, she would be alone forever. He always told Jasmin she'd never do better than him, and she realized she had internalized that message. But, Jasmin's friends reminded her, she deserved better. She was just as entitled to love and respect as anyone else.

Now that Jasmin had dug deep and found her negative core belief, she was determined to see things differently. That's what you'll learn to do in this chapter.

Revisit Your Goals

Look back at the goals you set in chapter 2. How do you think learning to identify and reshape your core beliefs might help you achieve those goals?

Identifying Your Negative Core Beliefs

Core beliefs are the general principles and assumptions that guide you through life. They can be positive: "Most people are good," or, "I can do anything I set my mind to," for example. But they can also be self-limiting, tricking your mind into seeing the world as darker and less full of possibility than it really is. Core beliefs have a number of potential origins, including childhood experiences, environmental factors, and your innate temperament. And while it can be helpful to determine where your core beliefs came from, you don't need to pinpoint their origins in order to identify and uproot them.

COMMON CORE BELIEFS

People with low self-confidence often find that one of the following core beliefs is at play. If one or more of the items on this list resonate with you, I'll show you how to delve deeper into these beliefs later in the chapter.

I don't belong. Being rejected by peers or even family at an early age can make you carry an "outsider" identity for years afterward. As an adult, you might avoid engaging with others for fear of rejection, or you might swing to the other extreme and become overly concerned with being the perfect group member.

The world is dangerous. This negative core belief leads to a lot of worrying and risk avoidance. If you believe there's evil or misfortune lurking around every corner, you're likely to restrict your activities and seek excessive reassurance to alleviate your anxiety. You also tend to overestimate the probability of negative outcomes and underestimate your ability to cope.

I am a failure/I'm not good enough. A persistent feeling of not measuring up can often be traced back to overcritical parents, bullying from class-mates, or a tendency to compare yourself to others. This belief can lead people to push themselves too hard to overcompensate. It also drives impostor syndrome, the constant feeling that you're a fraud and you'll be unmasked any day now. People who see themselves as failures can also be prone to avoidance or procrastination, which allows them to say, "I didn't fail; I never really tried."

I have to be perfect. A cousin of "I'm not good enough," this core belief also leads people to drive themselves until their health or relationships suffer. Perfectionists have unrealistically high expectations and tend to focus on their flaws and missteps. They may have trouble taking life less seriously and often have the sense that there is too little time.

LOOK FOR THEMES

Look through your records of your automatic negative thoughts. Do you notice any themes?

See if any of what you noted matches up with the list below. Check whether any of these beliefs *feel* correct to you, even if you understand intellectually that they are unrealistic.

- [ ] I'm not good enough.
- [ ] I can't get anything right.
- [ ] I'm worthless.
- [ ] I'm a failure.
- [ ] I am abnormal.
- [ ] I'm not wanted.
- [ ] I am unlovable.
- [ ] I don't fit in.
- [ ] I'm all alone.
- [ ] I'm not important.
- [ ] I'm not as good as other people.
- [ ] I'm sure to be rejected.
- [ ] I am weak.
- [ ] I don't measure up to others.
- [ ] I am unsuccessful.
- [ ] I can't handle anything.
- [ ] I'm a loser.
- [ ] I can't make a mistake.
- [ ] I have to be perfect.
- [ ] My needs are not important.
- [ ] I'm not a worthwhile person.
- [ ] Other theme I noticed: _____

FOLLOW THE PATH

"Following the path" of irrational thoughts is a process in which you ask yourself, or a therapist or trusted friend asks you, "What would happen then?"

Most of the employees in Claire's department were invited to a colleague's weekend baby shower. Claire kept hearing people talking about it, and she was hurt that she wasn't invited. She brought it up with her therapist, who asked simple questions to help Claire follow the path back to an untrue core belief.

They don't like me.

What would happen then? What does that mean?
I'll never have good friends.

What would happen then? What does that mean?
I'll never have a relationship.

What would happen then? What does that mean?
I'm unlovable.

Without following the chain of her thoughts, Claire never would have realized that her fixation on her coworker's baby shower really wasn't about the party itself. It was about a deep-down belief that she wasn't worthy of love or inclusion.

Try it yourself with one of the negative thoughts you noticed while monitoring your inner critic in chapter 5.

My thought:

_____

What would happen then? What does that mean?

_____

What would happen then? What does that mean?

_____

Repeat this process of questioning yourself until you arrive at what feels like the root: your negative core belief.

_____

_____

_____

DEVELOP A BETTER SENSE OF SELF

Knowing your own values and goals goes a long way toward developing a healthy sense of self, allowing you to be resilient after setbacks and resistant to pressure from those around you. But as you dig into your core beliefs, you might find there are ways you've set your authentic self aside in order to live by others' expectations. Here are some ideas to get in touch with who you really are.

Set boundaries. If you have trouble saying no, it's easy to end up doing a whole bunch of things that have nothing to do with what you love or value.

Get comfortable with being alone. Maybe you really want to see a certain movie or visit a certain city, but you just don't think anyone will go with you. Don't let that stop you!

Avoid comparison. Try to catch yourself when you feel like you don't measure up to someone else, and remember that we're all on different paths in life.

Know what motivates you. Maybe signing up for an 8 a.m. spin class just doesn't make you any more likely to exercise, and you know it. That's fine! Structure your life around what makes *you* stick with a goal, not what works for a friend.

Be a rebel. Now, you don't have to flout expectations all the time, or even most of the time. But if there's something everyone else is doing, and it just doesn't match up with what you believe in or care about, have the courage to go another way.

USE YOUR FEELINGS AS CLUES

Although much of the work of identifying and changing core beliefs involves using your mind, you must also allow your emotions to inform the process, or it will be incomplete. Change actually takes place in that "aha" moment when your feelings click with your thinking.

Unfortunately, many people hold mistaken ideas about emotions. Sometimes people are afraid of their feelings. Deep down they may have what seem to be very powerful and overwhelming feelings of fear, rage, or despair. They may assume they need to keep these feelings buried so that they aren't destroyed by them.

What about you? Look at this list below and check any that apply. (And don't worry; you're not alone if you check several, or even all, of these.)

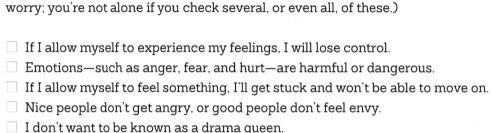

- [ ] If I allow myself to experience my feelings, I will lose control.
- [ ] Emotions—such as anger, fear, and hurt—are harmful or dangerous.
- [ ] If I allow myself to feel something, I'll get stuck and won't be able to move on.
- [ ] Nice people don't get angry, or good people don't feel envy.
- [ ] I don't want to be known as a drama queen.
- [ ] If others know how I really feel, they'll think I'm weak.

Although you may have been taught otherwise, feelings are important, not dangerous, and not inherently illogical. Your feelings likely developed for very specific reasons. For example, if you received harsh criticism as a child, you may be unable to allow yourself any feelings you perceive as risky—those that might force you to experience criticism or rejection again. You may be extremely vulnerable to the slightest complaint from a partner or coworker. This was a useful protective strategy when you were young and mostly defenseless. However, now that you're grown, these intense reactions can prove mysterious to yourself and others.

The key point is that an intense, seemingly out-of-the-blue emotional reaction is an important clue that a core belief is at work. If you can get a whiff of what's going on, it sets you up for that "aha" moment when you have a choice, a chance to react differently, and an opportunity to revise your belief.

The simple act of noting a feeling and naming it can be transformational. Ah, there's anger. Ah, there's fear. There's something about putting a label to a feeling that takes the edge away, making it softer and easier to handle. The lowered intensity of your reaction allows you to reassess your beliefs. For example, is it really true that nice people don't feel anger? Is it true that my anger will overtake me?

Establishing New Core Beliefs

How many times has life forced you to reevaluate what you believed? Maybe you were dead-set on believing your ex's new spouse was a terrible person, until they won you over by being a truly great stepparent to your kids. Maybe you were sure you would never learn to like Brussels sprouts, and then a good recipe changed your mind. Or maybe you had a more significant shift in beliefs, such as leaving your religion or switching political parties after you started to learn more about the world.

All of these belief shifts required a little bit of self-persuasion. You had to see, hear, or—in the case of the Brussels sprouts—taste the evidence in order to consider taking a new stance. The same is true for uprooting your negative core beliefs about yourself and supplanting them with positive ones. I'll show you how to look at your self-limiting beliefs from new angles until your mind starts to change.

CONSIDER YOUR PAST

You might roll your eyes at the idea of examining your childhood, but the truth is that negative core beliefs can often be traced back to your early days. Even when parents are trying their best, sometimes a mismatch in temperaments can leave a kid feeling left out or judged by the rest of the family. The same is true in peer groups. After you leave the nest, even if you find a supportive chosen family, you might hold on to untrue beliefs about yourself that formed in your childhood. For example, maybe you were an artistic child, but your parents discouraged you from pursuing that path because they didn't see it as sensible. Today, you might tell yourself that creativity is less valuable than making money or is incompatible with being a serious person. Those beliefs from your past are affecting your actions in the present.

Here's an exercise. Look at the list of core beliefs you identified earlier in this chapter. See if you can find messages in your past that echo those feelings, whether implicit or explicit. For instance, maybe your dad never showed up at your baseball games, making you think, "I'm not important," whether or not he ever said so. Or maybe your mother left the family when you were little, and now you think, "I'm not worthy of love." Whatever it is, let your feelings flow in the space provided.

LOOK FOR EVIDENCE

Beliefs come in pairs. If one of your internal messages is, "I'm not good enough," you can begin to starve that belief by feeding its benevolent twin, "I am good enough." Look for evidence to build up the good belief: the ways your contributions made a difference, the obstacles you overcame, the people who love and support you. Slowly, you'll begin to draw your mind's attention away from the flaws and failures that you mistakenly think disqualify you from your dreams.

Try it below.

My negative core belief:

The opposite, positive belief:

Evidence for the positive belief:

Review this list whenever you need a pick-me-up. But don't stop there. Keep bolstering the list of evidence with new experiences. This works especially well when your limiting belief says, "I can't." Maybe you think, "I'm just not athletic. My friends want me to join their recreational soccer league, but I know I'll embarrass myself." Well, why not try it? After a few weeks, you might prove yourself wrong. And then, forever after, you'll know that you're capable of far more than you might believe before you try.

CONDUCT MINI EXPERIMENTS

Think back to the science classes you took in school. Remember the steps for conducting an experiment? First, you state your hypothesis—in other words, what do you think will happen? Then, you design some type of procedure to test the hypothesis. Next, you record and examine the results to see if your hypothesis is supported or if alternative explanations should be considered. You can also use this approach to develop new core beliefs.

Kiara, recently divorced, was working on developing the confidence to do more things on her own. Over the years, she'd grown dependent on her partner for all her social needs. For example, she realized she had never been to a movie by herself, much less eaten in a restaurant alone. During one of our sessions, she talked about a documentary she really wanted to see, but said there was no way she'd have the nerve to go alone. When I asked her why, she said, "No one goes to the movies alone. It's all couples or groups of friends." When I pressed a bit further, we got to the belief that only losers go places alone.

I didn't think Kiara would simply listen to me if I told her I thought some people went to the movies alone. Instead, I asked her if she'd be willing to try a little experiment. We devised a plan whereby she arrived at the theater several minutes late for the movie she wanted to see. She didn't think she could tolerate standing in line or waiting in the lobby by herself. By going a little late, she could miss some of the crowds. After she had her ticket and was inside, she was to sit in the back row on an end, and she'd be free to leave after she collected her "data."

Kiara's job was to count the number of people sitting by themselves. If the light was such that she could notice anything about these people, she was also to jot down her observations. Did they look like losers? Were they acting like losers? Were they doing anything that called attention to themselves? Or were they just sitting there watching the movie?

When I saw Kiara for her next session, I crossed my fingers that there were in fact a few people there by themselves. Sure enough, Kiara had counted six people who were watching the movie alone. She laughed when I asked her if any of them looked like losers. She said, "I don't know. I got so into the movie I stopped paying attention to them." Kiara anticipated my next thought when she added, "I guess since I wasn't paying attention to them, no one would be paying attention to me."

This proved to be a powerful method to shift Kiara's belief and give her the confidence to start living again after her divorce.

FOCUS ON THE GOOD

Of course, humans are emotional creatures, and sometimes trying to be rational about your beliefs just doesn't work. That's when it's time to appeal to your feelings.

Focus again on the positive flip side of one of your negative beliefs. Think about a time when the positive belief really felt true, no matter how fleeting the feeling was. For instance, if your negative belief is, "I'm not good enough," recall a time when you did feel "good enough." Soak in that feeling for a few minutes, and remind yourself that you can and will feel that way again.

Allow yourself to accept new evidence of the good belief, even when you feel like dismissing it. Maybe you landed an interview for your dream job, and your instinct is to tell yourself, "Well, this is just a fluke. They'll never hire me." Instead of making that leap to negativity, take a moment to truly recognize and celebrate that the employer was impressed by your credentials and wants to meet you. Keeping your perceived flaws in perspective is key to recalibrating your belief system toward realistic, self-compassionate views.

"CONFIDENCE IS JUST ENTITLEMENT. ENTITLEMENT HAS GOTTEN A BAD RAP BECAUSE IT'S USED ALMOST EXCLUSIVELY FOR THE USELESS CHILDREN OF THE RICH . . . BUT ENTITLEMENT IN AND OF ITSELF ISN'T SO BAD. ENTITLEMENT IS SIMPLY THE BELIEF THAT YOU DESERVE SOMETHING."

—MINDY KALING

One of the fundamental beliefs underlying confidence is, "My worth as a person is equal to everyone else's." That doesn't mean you don't have to work for what you want, and it certainly doesn't mean life divides up its rewards evenly. But it does mean you have the same right as anyone else to stand up for yourself, pursue your dreams, enjoy your life, and make a difference in the way that's most meaningful to you.

Sometimes it's almost impossible to picture yourself up there with those you admire most. You think, "What so-and-so does is wonderful, but me, I could *never* do that. I just don't have the right stuff." When messages like that run through your head, don't just let them pass. Stop them. Question them. What is the "right stuff"?

Maybe you think you're not suited for a role in life because you don't fit a certain mold: You don't come from the "right" background, you don't run in the "right" crowd, you don't look the "right" way, or you don't have the "right" personality. You're counting yourself out before you even start, creating limitations that might prove not to exist at all if you tested them.

To be sure, some dreams do expire. A 50-year-old who's never played baseball isn't going to make it to the majors. And even when the potential for success is there, breaking the mold can be really tough—ask anyone who's been the only woman or person of color in the room, for instance. But don't be the one who rejects your dream. Be the one who continues to push for it even when other people tell you that you'll never get there. With hard work, you will.

THE FEAR FACTOR: WORKING WITH YOUR BELIEFS

Questioning beliefs that have long seemed like fundamental truths is scary stuff. Earlier in this chapter, when you worked on finding evidence to support positive beliefs, you might have felt a little overwhelmed. That's because a negative belief can be a nice excuse to stay inside your comfort zone: "Well, I'll never succeed, so there's no point in trying!" When you start to let go of those beliefs, you might suddenly feel vulnerable. Now there's no excuse not to try, and trying might mean failing.

Jot down any fears or trepidation you felt while working through this chapter.

_____

_____

_____

_____

It's natural to resist adopting positive beliefs because you're afraid of getting burned once you "buy in." But your negative core beliefs are hurting you, too. They keep you trapped, telling you the lie that no risk is ever worthwhile. Ask yourself whether you'd really prefer to spend your life locked in a tower like Rapunzel, avoiding risks but never knowing what it feels like to reach your full potential.

Now, you won't uproot your negative core beliefs overnight. Some days you'll feel pretty hopeful, and on others, all the old self-limiting stories will creep back in. That's perfectly normal. Remember to look at the big picture and see all the progress you've made. Then, get back out there and try again.

Chapter Takeaways

Now you're well on your way to reshaping your view of yourself and the world in a way that allows you to walk through life with greater confidence that things will go well for you. In the next chapter, you'll zero in on your fears. Using the exposure therapy tools you learned about in chapter 1, you'll set a plan to begin conquering scary situations, one small step at a time.

ACTION ITEMS

Here are some specific actions you can take to implement the lessons and ideas you learned in this chapter:

1. Look over old journals or letters from 10 or 20 years ago. Were there any self-limiting beliefs you had back then that you came to find out weren't true? Think about how worthwhile it was to prove yourself wrong.

2. Create a visual reminder of evidence of the positive beliefs you're working to build. This could be as simple as putting photos on your fridge that remind you of goals you've reached and people who love you. Or, if you want to put in a little more time, you could make a whole collage reminding you that you are loved, capable, big-hearted, and so on.

3. Read a book or watch a movie about someone who pushed past limiting beliefs (their own or others') to achieve something great. Some suggestions: *Sisters in Law: How Sandra Day O'Connor and Ruth Bader Ginsburg Went to the Supreme Court and Changed the World* by Linda Hirshman; *The Story of My Life* by Helen Keller; *Legally Blonde* by Amanda Brown (also a movie and a musical); and *The Blind Side*, written and directed by John Lee Hancock.

4. Think about the people in your life who tend to support positive beliefs and see if you can spend more time with them. Similarly, if there are people who

consistently make you feel negatively about yourself or the world, try to limit your time with them.

5. Consider how the news and entertainment you consume might be affecting your beliefs. For example, if you're trying to stop thinking danger is lurking around every corner, you might try cutting back on true-crime dramas and TV news.

CHAPTER SEVEN

FACE YOUR FEARS

· · · · · · · ·

"FEAR KEEPS US FOCUSED ON THE PAST OR WORRIED ABOUT THE FUTURE. IF WE CAN ACKNOWLEDGE OUR FEAR, WE CAN REALIZE THAT RIGHT NOW WE ARE OKAY. RIGHT NOW, TODAY, WE ARE STILL ALIVE, AND OUR BODIES ARE WORKING MARVELOUSLY. OUR EYES CAN STILL SEE THE BEAUTIFUL SKY. OUR EARS CAN STILL HEAR THE VOICES OF OUR LOVED ONES."

—THICH NHAT HANH

You can tell yourself, "There's nothing to be afraid of." But words aren't enough. Anyone who's ever tried to tell a frightened three-year-old that there are no monsters in the closet knows the futility of mere words. You have to *show* the child it's safe by shining a flashlight in the closet, poking all around, encouraging the child to look in, and so on. For beliefs to fully change, they must be disproved on a very basic, gut level.

That's what we'll do in this chapter. We'll shine a light on what scares you and give you practical tools and strategies to look fear in the eye, so you can move forward with greater self-confidence. I'll walk you through it step-by-step; remember from chapter 2 that I'm not going to throw you into the deep end of the pool not knowing how to swim. Also, I think you'll find that with the strategies you've gathered over the past few chapters, facing your fears will be easier than you imagine.

Facing Fear

Remember that fear is a natural and normal part of our evolutionary heritage. We need a fear response so we know not to run out into traffic or put our hand on a hot stove. Of course, problems arise when our fears are unfounded or exaggerated. Learning to face our fears can be powerful, especially if it's done in a systematic way, such as with exposure therapy.

HOW IT WORKS

I typically describe exposure therapy to people using a lighthearted example to diminish any anxiety they may have about the process. You may remember a cartoon called *Rugrats*, which aired from 1991 through 2004. The show addressed common childhood experiences through humor and understanding.

In the episode "The Slide," the ever fretful Chuckie Finster longs to go down the slide and have fun like all the other kids at the park. But when he looks up, the slide appears menacing. His perpetual nemesis, Angelica, makes fun of him and calls him a "scaredy cat." Fortunately, Chuckie has a good friend in Tommy Pickles. Tommy takes Chuckie to the smartest kid on the block, Susie, who agrees to help. Under Susie's guidance, the neighborhood kids help Chuckie face his fears by gradually exposing him to heights, going back and forth in a tire swing, having a fan blowing hard in his face, and traveling fast in a wagon. As he gets used to the physical sensations connected to heights and moving at a high rate of speed, Susie instructs him to tell himself repeatedly, "I'm a big, brave dog!"

Of course, the episode ends with Chuckie triumphantly climbing up the slide and enjoying the trip back down. When the other kids ask how he overcame his fears, he answers, "I just did. That's all."

WHY IT WORKS

One way exposure works is through a process called *habituation*. This means that the more you become accustomed to something, the less it feels like a big deal. It's more like a habit that is simply a part of your life. Habituation is at work when you no longer notice the sound of leaf blowers in the fall, or that rattling refrigerator ceases to annoy you.

Another way exposure therapy works is by helping you shift your expectations about what will happen in a given situation. You learn that the chances of something awful happening are pretty slim, and if something awful did happen, you could cope. Comments I hear from people after they successfully complete exposure therapy include:

- "I can function when I'm feeling anxious."
- "Anxiety goes away with time. It doesn't last forever."
- "I still don't like anxiety, but I know it's not going to kill me."
- "I'm stronger than I thought I was."

CREATING A HIERARCHY

Merima immigrated from Bosnia nearly five years ago with her husband, Esad. Esad works at a grocery store and they have two children, who are now in school. Merima learned to drive about a year after coming to the United States, but she didn't like it. Esad assured her she was a safe and competent driver, but she still felt anxious about her abilities and avoided it whenever possible. She told him she didn't have much need to drive when the children were young and at home. Esad took her to run errands on the weekends. However, now the kids were in school and she yearned to become more independent. She wanted to volunteer at the children's school and be able to run her own errands during the week.

Merima worked with a counselor through a nearby international center who knew about exposure therapy. Together they constructed a hierarchy: a detailed plan to get Merima driving again. She already knew how to drive, but she needed to gain confidence in her abilities and get over her fear.

When creating a hierarchy, the trick is to break your fear into a series of steps, with the first few steps being mildly challenging and later steps increasing in difficulty. It's a list that is rank-ordered by the amount of distress each step would lead to if you completed it.

Below you'll see Merima's exposure hierarchy.

Mild-Challenge Activities
(Anxiety level would rise to no more than a 3 on a 10-point scale, with 10 being the worst possible anxiety.)

Sit in driver's seat of car.
Pull out of my driveway.
Drive around the block with husband.
Drive around the block alone.

Moderate-Challenge Activities
(Anxiety level would rise to a level of 4 to 7, with 10 being the worst possible anxiety.)

Drive in the neighborhood for 10 minutes with husband.
Drive in neighborhood for 10 minutes alone.
Turn left on a residential street with husband.
Turn left on a residential street alone.

(Anxiety level would rise to a level of 8 to 10, with 10 being the worst possible anxiety.)

Drive on city streets in light traffic with husband.
Drive on city streets in light traffic alone.
Drive on city streets in moderate traffic with husband.
Drive on city streets in moderate traffic alone.

Notice how Merima's plan starts with a small challenge, sitting in the car. You might think, "That is so easy!" But for Merima, this was enough to elicit some mild anxiety, so it was a good starting point. Starting with small steps not only maximizes her chance for success but also motivates her to continue when the exposures get a little tougher.

Use the My Exposure Hierarchy form to write out your own plan. Remember, this is your plan, your goals. Notice that Merima didn't have on her hierarchy anything about highway driving. She may decide to add that later, but for now, she doesn't see that as crucial to her independence. Aim to strike a balance, making a plan that will help you accomplish your goals without needlessly overwhelming you.

My Exposure Hierarchy
Mild-Challenge Activities

Moderate-Challenge Activities

High-Challenge Activities

HOW TO CARRY OUT YOUR EXPOSURES

1. Start with the first item on your hierarchy, one in the mild-challenge range.
2. Enter the situation and carry out the exposure (for example, Merima sits in the driver's seat of the car).
3. Your anxiety level will start to rise. This is a sign that the exposure is working. Allow yourself to feel the sensations, and realize that anxiety won't harm you; you can tolerate it.
4. You can use your breathing techniques and a coping statement to help you, but you don't want to let them become distractions. The goal is to learn that anxiety isn't dangerous, and you can't do that if you don't let yourself fully experience the symptoms.
5. Stay in the situation until your anxiety level starts to decline. If you leave the situation when your anxiety level is too high, it reinforces the fear. The general idea is that you want to remain in the situation long enough to know that anxiety doesn't last indefinitely and that you can handle the situation.
6. Repeat the item until you have the sense that you could do it again without major difficulty. This will likely require many practice sessions. Then you can move to the next item on the hierarchy.
7. Write a record of your exposure sessions on the My Exposure Log.

Note: If you find that any particular exposure session isn't going well—perhaps your anxiety is getting higher than you thought it would when you created your hierarchy—it is okay to occasionally stop the session early. You don't want to make this a habit, but you do want to feel in control of the pace of your progress. Nothing is lost; simply start again on an easier item and work your way back up.

Once you get going, you'll likely find that it progressively takes less time to complete an exposure session. This is because you take with you what you've learned from one session to another. For example, by the time Merima got to her medium-challenge exposures of driving in the neighborhood, her body had already calmed down and she wasn't nearly as shaky behind the wheel as she was simply backing out of the driveway.

My Exposure Log

What I Did	Challenge Level (Mild, Moderate, or High)	Time Spent	Anxiety Level at Start (1-10)	Anxiety Level at Finish (1-10)

CONFIDENCE CRUTCHES

Many people employ habits to bolster self-confidence that work in the short run but backfire in the long run. Psychologists call these *safety behaviors* or *partial avoidance behaviors*. In other words, someone may go into a feared situation but rely on a crutch to control the resulting anxiety. See if you relate to any of these examples:

- Sitting in the back of the class or conference room, where you won't have to interact.
- Going to a party only if you can drink ahead of time.
- Using substances excessively to cope with feared situations (self-medicating).
- Never arriving early for a meeting so you can avoid small talk.
- Avoiding eye contact by mindlessly fidgeting with your phone.
- Engaging in excessive research or overpreparing to make sure nothing goes wrong.
- Always having a companion with you.
- Keeping your eyes glued to your notes when you're giving a speech.

The problem with these behaviors is that you think nothing bad happened because you used the crutch. You don't have a chance to prove to yourself that you could succeed on your own.

Other tips for successful exposure therapy:

Practice frequently. If you let too much time go by between exposure sessions, you can lose motivation and momentum.

Minimize distractions. As I mentioned above, it's fine to use your breathing techniques and a simple coping statement, such as, "I can tolerate anxiety; it's not that bad." But if you find yourself engaging in a lot of other rituals that distract you from fully engaging with the exposure item, you're not getting the full benefit.

Give yourself credit. No matter how one particular exposure session goes, you deserve to feel good about your efforts. Just like Chuckie, you're a big, brave dog!

IMAGINAL EXPOSURE

Sometimes you may benefit from imaginal exposure, a variation of habituating yourself to your fears in real life. The principles are the same; the only exception is that you'll carry out your exposures in your mind. Imaginal exposure can side-swipe some problems people may encounter in traditional exposure therapy. For example, what if Merima became extremely anxious simply sitting in a car? You could break it down even further, having her approach the car, then stand 10 feet away, and so on. Or she could desensitize herself by imagining the scene first. Typically, you write out a brief script, including as many details as possible about the situation, especially details about the things you fear will happen. You include any troubling physical sensations, thoughts you may experience, and what you imagine other people's reactions will be, if applicable. Once you get comfortable doing the exposure in your mind, you can switch to doing it in real life.

Learn to Handle Fear of Failure

One of the best confidence-building strategies is to treat mistakes as learning experiences. I know it sounds like something you'd see on a sappy motivational poster, but there's no better way to create a rich and fulfilling life than to get good at failing. So what are the keys to failing well?

Although intellectually we know failing can prove to be a learning experience, it's still no fun. When a situation doesn't go as planned, what's your first instinct? Check any or all that apply.

☐ I typically look for someone or something to blame.
☐ I tend to blame myself.
☐ I avoid thinking about what happened.
☐ I overeat, overspend, overuse substances, binge-watch TV, and so on.

It's natural to want to avoid uncomfortable feelings. By now you probably remember that avoidance leads to more suffering. In addition, avoiding your feelings can actually lead to less effective processing of the experience, meaning you don't learn as much from it.

It takes bravery not to numb out—to feel the immediacy and rawness of the experience. And sure, sometimes it makes sense to take a break and engage in a distraction if you're overwhelmed. That's just good self-care. But don't stay away too long; know when it's time to come home to your feelings.

DON'T LABEL YOURSELF AS A FAILURE

The fact that you made a mistake does not mean you are a failure as a human being. Making a mistake is a specific behavior or event. Telling yourself that you are a failure is a very global self-judgment. Notice this thought progression:

I made several mistakes on an exam.
I failed the exam.
I am a failure.

Instead, a healthier way of looking at this would be:

I made several mistakes on the exam.
I failed the exam.
I need to talk to the professor and make a plan.

Think back to a time you "failed" at something. Can you rewrite the story so that you don't condemn yourself as a human being?

KEEP YOUR SENSE OF HUMOR

A few months ago, my husband attended a workshop for psychologists on how to handle giving expert testimony in court. Most people become quite anxious at the thought of testifying in court, and one of the goals of the presentation was to familiarize the audience with how to handle questions that might trip them up. The presenter, a distinguished forensic psychologist who had decades of court testimony under his belt, said that he's still asked questions that he has no idea how to answer. Previously serious in nature, the presenter threw up his arms and exclaimed, "What can I say? I'm a flawed human being!" The nervous psychologists all laughed with relief. I thought this was such a great story. Of course, even experts are human. It's become one of my go-to reminders to myself when I'm feeling anxious about a mistake: "Hey, I'm a flawed human being!" I tell myself this, and then I can quickly move on to assess what, if anything, I need to do to rectify the mistake.

Set Yourself Up to Win

Tackling your fears as a means of developing your self-confidence is a big undertaking, but there are a few important things you can do to improve your chances of success from the start. Here are a few tips that will help you use your own motivational tendencies to your advantage.

DEVELOP GOOD HABITS

Many of the techniques in this chapter require dedication. Developing effective habits can pay big dividends in making your hard work pay off. One way to develop any habit is called *habit stacking*. The formula goes like this:

After I _____, I will _____.

For example,

After I brush my teeth, I will meditate.

Think of a habit associated with this chapter that you'd like to incorporate into your day. Use the formula above and write out your plan.

After I _____, I will _____.

You pair an activity you do without thought with the new habit you want to develop. With consistency, the association will become strong and you'll naturally move from one activity to another with more ease.

Another aspect you can add to habit stacking is chaining. This means that you try not to "break the chain" by skipping a day. For example, you might mark on your calendar every day you do the desired habit and try not to skip any day. This can be quite motivating for some people. However, for others, if they miss a day, they may feel they've blown it and quit. Know yourself and decide whether or not this tip will work for you.

Another important aspect of developing good habits is scheduling. Make note of any items in this chapter that you want to include in your schedule and write them down, whether on a paper calendar, your phone's calendar app, or any other scheduling software you use. Most experts will tell you to do your hardest tasks in the morning, as willpower fades and energy dwindles throughout the day. But if you're not a morning person, this may not be the best timing for you.

One last tip is to set up your environment to support your goals. For example, if you're trying to incorporate yoga into your routine, have your yoga mat set up where you will see it. You can also try pairing it with something you enjoy. I've known people who take their morning coffee and simply sit on their yoga mat. After they've enjoyed their coffee, they are already on the mat, and more often than not, they do their yoga routine. Often, the hardest part of any habit is simply starting.

CHANGE YOUR STRESS MIND-SET

When you tackle a new project, face a feared situation, or wade out of your comfort zone, your body is going to register it as a stressor, even though you may be doing it to build self-confidence. We've been bombarded with messages that stress is bad for you: It can cause all sorts of health problems from heart disease to cancer, not to mention anxiety, depression, and just plain old burnout. A book by psychologist Kelly McGonigal has called these long-held beliefs about stress into question. In *The Upside of Stress*, she shares scores of research studies that show how stress can benefit you if you have the right mind-set.

According to the research, stress usually indicates that something that matters to you is at stake. Of course, stress can feel terrible if you view the situation as a threat, even when the situation isn't life or death. Take moving for instance. You might say to yourself, "I'm stressed about moving to a new city. If we don't find a good neighborhood and make a lot of new friends, I'll be miserable!" But if you think back to the values work you did in chapter 2, you can see how the stress is signaling an opportunity to buckle down, use all your resources, and rise to the occasion.

First, use your mindfulness skills to notice the stress without judging it. Next, ask yourself what's at stake that matters to you. How does it tie into your values? Maybe the move will be a perfect opportunity to live your values of providing a better life for your family and contributing to a community of like-minded people. Keeping that values-driven answer in mind, tell yourself the stressful situation is a *challenge*, not a threat. Remind yourself that you have everything you need to prepare for the move and establish yourself successfully.

I encourage you to use effective stress management techniques, such as deep breathing and realistic self-talk, to face any of your confidence challenges. But use these techniques to help you feel more comfortable as you pursue your valued goals—not in a fearful attempt to get rid of stress because stress is bad for you.

SEEK OUT SUPPORT

The type of social support your ancestors may have known—one in which bonds were formed based on kinship, geography, or religious ideology—may not work for you. Although these types of bonds had many strengths, they also had weaknesses, such as rigidity and exclusivity. In the past, if you didn't fit a particular mold, you may have been ostracized from the group.

Nowadays, you may have to deliberately develop a support system. This is your chance to gather your own unique group of people to walk this path with you. If you're an introvert, this may sound daunting. You may be thinking to yourself, "I can't go up to someone and ask them to be part of my support system!" Don't worry, I don't expect you to do that. What you can do is be open to opportunities that naturally arise and be willing to risk putting yourself in new situations to meet people.

Look for people who can serve different roles in your life:

- ☐ Someone who can pump you up when you're feeling down.
- ☐ Someone to provide emotional support and a shoulder to cry on.
- ☐ Someone to give you honest feedback in a helpful way.
- ☐ Someone who can provide practical information and support.

Add any others you think are important:

- ☐ ....
- ☐ ....
- ☐ ....
- ☐ ....

Prepare, Prepare, Prepare

No one doubts that preparation underlies any successful endeavor. Whether it's giving a speech or playing in a band, you simply can't perform well without consistent and deliberate practice. Here's a game plan for honing your practice sessions and developing self-confidence:

1. Determine what skill or set of skills you need to practice. If you're concerned about your social skills, ask yourself, "What is it that's missing?" Do you find you're lacking in topics to spark conversation? Or do you have plenty to talk about, but you come across as expressionless or aloof, leaving others to wonder if you're interested and paying attention? In that case, you need to practice nonverbal communication skills. If you're preparing for a presentation, maybe you most need to work on an engaging opening or how to handle a Q and A session.
2. Experiment with the new skill. Sticking with the nonverbal communication example, experimenting might mean practicing in front of a mirror or having yourself videotaped. Some people benefit from exaggerating their expressions at first, later finding a natural middle ground. Although it might be a little intimidating, asking someone for feedback might help.
3. Use visualization to prepare for the best-case scenario, the worst-case scenario, and the most likely scenario. Imagining an undesirable outcome and realizing you'd survive provides good stress inoculation.
4. Practice in the actual setting if possible. For example, if you're giving a presentation, can you get into the venue ahead of time to scope out the setup?

5. It is likely that the skills you need to practice will change over time. As you master one area, a new one will emerge as needing focus.

6. Once you've prepared, let go of the outcome.

Be Patient with Yourself

Personal growth takes more time than we anticipate, and most of us aren't taught to develop patience. Marketing and advertising are partly to blame: We're sold on the idea that the quick fix is the norm. Even books such as this one, in an attempt to present things as simply as possible, may unwittingly give the impression that change is a neat and tidy process. In reality, when I'm working with someone on exposure therapy, we may refine their hierarchy multiple times. Unexpected setbacks occur.

Keep in mind, too, that most of us spiral through the same issues throughout our lives. This is not meant to discourage you but to normalize and validate the idea that life is hard. We're often presented with similar challenges over and over. Each time we confront our issues and fears, we hopefully progress, but we're never really done. Learning, growing, and changing are lifelong processes.

Patience can be cultivated in small situations in everyday life:

- When you're stuck in a long line at the grocery store.
- When traffic is not moving as fast as you'd like.
- When your child is taking "too long" to put on shoes.
- When you're waiting for an email response.

When you're in a situation that's trying your patience, consider it practice for bigger challenges. Use it as an opportunity to do a brief mindfulness practice. Make eye contact with someone and realize you're in this together. Mentally run through a list of things for which you're grateful. And if you're still frustrated, be kind to yourself. Allow yourself to feel the frustration, notice where you're tensing in your body, and try to soften those muscles just a tiny bit.

Make a Commitment

Facing your fears can initially be daunting, but by now you've learned some doable ways to make it manageable. Still, it can be easy to get sidetracked with your busy day-to-day life. Making a commitment can strengthen your resolve and formalize your efforts. To begin, remind yourself of the benefits of facing your fears. Merima, the Bosnian immigrant with the driving phobia you met earlier, wrote the following benefits of being able to drive:

- I'll be more independent. I can go places without asking my husband to take me.
- I'll model for my children that they can deal with challenges head-on.
- I'll feel proud of myself for accomplishing this goal.

Remind yourself of the benefits of facing your fear:

Next, anticipate what might get in the way of keeping your commitment. Possibilities include emotions, negative self-talk, poor habits, or lack of support. Jot down any potential obstacles you might encounter. After that, write down a potential solution. For example:

Potential obstacle: **No time without the kids around to practice my exposures.**
Possible solution: **Offer to exchange childcare with a neighborhood mom.**

Now you grab a pen and try it out.

Potential obstacle:

Possible solution:

_____

Potential obstacle:

_____

Possible solution:

_____

Potential obstacle:

_____

Possible solution:

_____

Now, write down a realistic commitment that takes into account the benefits you've listed as well as any potential obstacles. For example, you might commit to practicing your exposures three times a week for 30 minutes at a time. Or you might commit more generally to practicing the exercises in this book for 30 minutes a day.

My realistic commitment is:

_____

_____

_____

_____

_____

"THE BIGGEST COMMITMENT YOU MUST KEEP IS YOUR COMMITMENT TO YOURSELF."

—NEALE DONALD WALSCH

THE FEAR FACTOR: FACING YOUR FEARS

It goes without saying that facing your fears is bound to bring on a lot of, well, fear! But it's important to sort through any resistance you felt while familiarizing yourself with the concepts in this chapter. For instance, maybe you've had a bad experience with a family member or friend who thought the best way to "cure" you of a fear was to force you to face it all at once. Even though that's not the same as the gradual exposure you learned about in this chapter, you may be turned off of any strategy involving confronting your fears.

Or maybe you recognized your own habits in the sidebar on confidence crutches (page 130), but you just don't know how you're supposed to get through an overwhelming situation without your safety behavior. Write out some of your fears or hesitation about implementing this chapter's advice in your own life.

_____

_____

_____

_____

_____

_____

If you're not enthusiastic about jumping right into exposure therapy, that's perfectly fine. Remember that you can start out with imaginal exposure. You also might consider seeking the help of a trained psychologist who can offer additional strategies and accountability as you work through your exposure hierarchy. Finally, know that although exposure therapy can feel daunting at the beginning, as you complete the first steps of your hierarchy, your confidence will grow by leaps and bounds. The momentum you gain early on will make the more anxiety-producing steps much easier than they seem now.

Chapter Takeaways

Congratulations! You now have a toolbox full of strategies to boost your self-confidence, and I'm willing to bet you have already started approaching your life a little differently. Maybe you've begun making small talk with other parents at school pickup, or putting your hat in the ring for opportunities you didn't think were worth pursuing before. A little bit of knowledge goes a long way, but now it's up to you to continue carrying on the practices you've learned in this book. In the next chapter, I'll teach you how to make confidence a lifelong habit.

ACTION ITEMS

Here are some specific actions you can take to implement the lessons and ideas you learned in this chapter:

1. If social situations are some of your biggest confidence challenges, visit psychologist Ellen Hendriksen's website: www.ellenhendriksen.com /mountains-to-molehills-challenge. She has compiled a long list of low-risk challenges for the socially anxious, including ways to practice being the center of attention and talking about yourself.

2. If you feel comfortable doing so, tell a friend or family member about your exposure hierarchy. Ask them to make sure you practice frequently and to help you celebrate when you master something on your list.

3. It may sound funny, but if you're struggling with a fear of failure, try making mistakes on purpose. Trip in public or pronounce a word wrong in a noticeable way. You'll likely find that the ensuing awkwardness isn't as bad as you feared.

4. Search for "failure résumés" online. You'll find scores of successful people who have published lists of the schools that rejected them, companies they started that went bust, and jobs they did not get. As you'll see, failures are not what define a person; they are merely a by-product of putting oneself out there.

5. Set a goal to kick your confidence crutches to the curb for a while. Go a week without fiddling with your phone in any social settings, or arrive early to all of your meetings and chat with your colleagues.

CHAPTER EIGHT

MOVING FORWARD

· · · · · · · ·

> "ONE'S DESTINATION IS NEVER A PLACE, BUT RATHER
> A NEW WAY OF LOOKING AT THINGS."
>
> —HENRY MILLER

Improving your self-confidence isn't a "one-and-done" kind of deal. It's something you'll have to keep practicing, and you're sure to encounter ups and downs along the way. Some days will go all wrong. You'll make embarrassing mistakes, you won't get your point across, people will be rude, and you might just want to go home and pull the covers over your head.

But when those days inevitably come, remember all the great things you're striving toward. Building confidence leads to less fear and anxiety, greater motivation, more resilience, better relationships, and a stronger sense of your authentic self. You're not the sort of person who would give all that up just because of a few setbacks—you haven't come this far just to turn back! You know by now that progress is made up of small steps. Even when you feel like you're going backward, you can always come back to basics and get yourself back on track.

PUTTING IT ALL TOGETHER

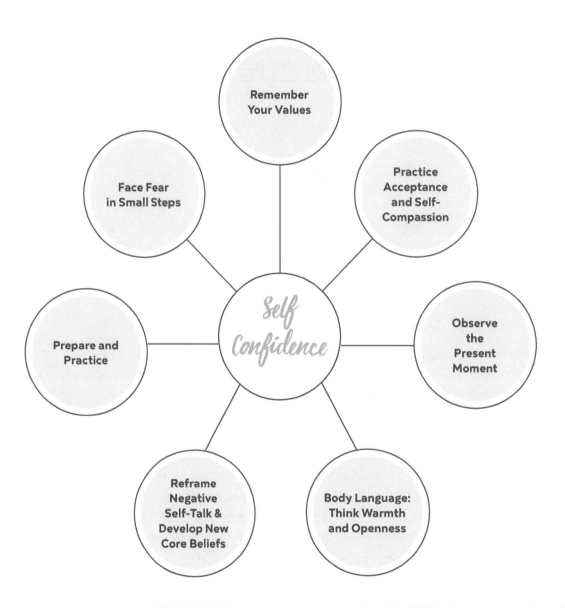

- Remember Your Values
- Practice Acceptance and Self-Compassion
- Observe the Present Moment
- Body Language: Think Warmth and Openness
- Reframe Negative Self-Talk & Develop New Core Beliefs
- Prepare and Practice
- Face Fear in Small Steps

Self Confidence

Stay in the Moment

Confidence comes from action, and you can take action only in the present. You already know that replaying your past mistakes thousands of times—far past the point where you've gleaned any useful insight about how to improve—keeps you from action. The same is true for worrying about what could go wrong in the future.

Although I hope you're finishing this book energized and ready to pursue your goals, you don't want to be so busy chasing your next accomplishment that you lose track of all the wonderful things happening right here in the present moment. When you find yourself time traveling to the past or future, review what you learned about mindfulness in chapter 4. You can also refer to the Resources section (page 153) to build your mindfulness skills.

Develop Long-Term Goals

The first step in developing long-term goals is getting a sense of the progress you've made. In chapter 1, you completed a Self-Confidence Scale (page 18). Take some time now to do it again, using a separate sheet of paper or a pen with a different color. I'm betting that if you've made a good faith effort at trying even some of the exercises in this book, your answers will reflect improved self-confidence. Note any observations you have about items that have changed and those that haven't.

In chapter 2, you set confidence goals for yourself in a number of life areas, such as career and family. Review the goals you set for yourself. Use the space below to note progress you've made. Try not to minimize how far you've come.

Oftentimes, after you've learned skills such as those in this book and get a taste of success, you'll notice other areas of your life where you could apply them. Remember the question I asked you in the beginning of the book: What would you do if you had all the confidence you wanted? Dare to imagine what other goals you might set for yourself.

The information you've gathered by retaking the Self-Confidence Scale and reviewing the goals from chapter 2 will help you plan your long-term goals. I've found it helpful to break them into time frames.

In the next month, I will:

In the next three to six months, I will:

In the next year, I will:

You may be surprised by the power of the simple act of putting your goals in writing and regularly reviewing them to make sure you're on track. You'll likely find that you're much more alert to potential opportunities and connections around you, just because you've made a written commitment to yourself to improve.

Accept Setbacks

Progress is frequently not linear. We make some strides, then hit a bump in the road. I don't expect you to jump for joy when you experience a setback. But after your initial gut reaction of getting angry about the problem or feeling disappointed, step back and ask yourself, "What can I learn here? What opportunities are hidden behind this obstacle?" Remember, you've gathered many skills throughout this book, skills that can help you cope with whatever lapse you encounter. When you hit a bump in the road, at least that means you're going somewhere.

I've included a worksheet you can use when you're dealing with some type of setback or obstacle in your self-confidence journey. It incorporates many of the skills we've used in this workbook.

Turning Obstacles into Opportunities

Situation:

Thought (What I'm telling myself):

Feelings (Resulting emotions):

_____

Probability of this occurring (How likely is it that what I'm thinking will actually happen?):

_____

Consequences if this occurs (How bad would it be?):

_____

Coping statement (What can I say to myself that is more realistic, more encouraging?):

_____

Action(s) I will take:

_____

Opportunity (How I can learn or grow by dealing with this):

_____

_____

WHAT IF IT'S MORE THAN A SETBACK?

What if you find your confidence sinking to an all-time low, despite your best efforts to follow the advice in this book? First of all, know that it's not your fault. You're brave to acknowledge that you're struggling. Please reach out to someone you trust and let them know how you're feeling. Talking with someone often helps you get back on track more quickly than you'd expect. If there is no one in your immediate community who can fulfill this role, find yourself a good mental health care professional. This is often a good idea in general when dealing with

DON'T LET SETBACKS STOP YOU

Review these tips when you encounter obstacles in your confidence journey. I'm sure you'll notice several harken back to concepts we've previously covered. It often takes reading things several times before we get it.

Expect setbacks. Change takes time and often requires frequent attempts. For example, most smokers require five to seven attempts before they finally quit. Were these attempts failures or part of their eventual success?

Check your stress level. An increase in physical or mental stress may be the reason you're struggling.

Practice self-care. Make self-care activities a priority by writing them down, almost like a policy.

Keep at it. If your plan involves specific activities—keeping a thought diary or practicing mindfulness—don't stop, even if you're doing well. Sometimes it's the good times, not the stressful ones, that take you off guard.

Recommit. Remind yourself of your goals and what you care deeply about. Recommit yourself to activities aligned with your values.

Remember you're human. We're all imperfect; it's part of being human. Remind yourself that setbacks happen to everyone.

Laugh when you can. Nurturing your sense of humor can be a great asset in embracing the ups and downs of life.

Seek out support. If you're feeling badly about "screwing up," your first instinct may be to hide in a hole. But this is exactly the time you need to reach out.

Give yourself credit. Remind yourself of the steps you've taken, regardless of how small they might seem to you.

Begin again. You don't have to wait until tomorrow or Monday to start doing the right thing. You can make the choice to honor your intentions in the very next moment.

self-confidence issues; while many of your loved ones may be capable of holding space for you to vent and process, they may not have the capacity to help you to get back up from the bottom. The Resources section (page 153) can help you find a mental health professional. You, as much as anyone else, deserve confidence and the peace and happiness that go with it, and a caring mental health practitioner can truly work wonders to get you to that place.

CONTINUE YOUR PRACTICE

Confidence is a little like a muscle: If you don't keep up with your exercises, you might find your skills weakening. Take some time to review the notes you've added to this workbook. What are the practices that you benefited from the most? For instance, did you find diaphragmatic breathing to be a helpful tool in calming your body? Are you still practicing and implementing this skill, or have you let this lapse? What about keeping track of your thoughts? Are you still keeping a thought diary? You don't have to do this every single day, but it's good to do it periodically so you can watch for faulty thinking patterns creeping back in. Are you still challenging yourself to face feared situations?

Use this time to design your own confidence tool kit by going through the book, chapter by chapter, and noting which skills, techniques, and ideas you want to focus on in the future. Write them down here, then rank them in terms of helpfulness.

A final suggestion is to set a weekly check-in time to revisit this workbook. Make it an enjoyable time you look forward to. Make yourself a cup of tea or another favorite beverage, and turn on some music that puts you in a positive frame of mind. Reread sections you found particularly helpful, and make notes of areas you want to focus on in the coming week.

THE WORLD NEEDS A CONFIDENT YOU

> "WITH THE REALIZATION OF ONE'S OWN POTENTIAL AND SELF-CONFIDENCE IN ONE'S ABILITY, ONE CAN BUILD A BETTER WORLD."
>
> —DALAI LAMA

Think about someone who has made a big difference in your life, whether they know it or not. Maybe it's a friend or partner who makes you smile when you need it most. Maybe it's a songwriter whose music really speaks to you and gets you through tough times. Or maybe it's a leader in your community or from history whose message, vision, and commitment inspire you to keep going.

Now imagine a different world—one in which that person decided not to be seen at all. Imagine that your partner never had the courage to ask you on a date, figuring the risk of rejection was too high. Imagine that your favorite songwriter never released an album, deciding their music just wasn't any good. And imagine the inspirational leader never had the courage to stand up for the principles that are so dear to you.

Nearly everything you find beautiful or enjoyable in life exists because someone else decided to put it there for you. They likely felt nagging self-doubt or perhaps near-paralyzing fear about what they were doing, but their values carried them through. They stepped out the door and braved the attention and criticism for their efforts, and the world is a better place as a result.

You can be just as brave as your heroes. With the tools in this book, you are ready to stop hiding your light under a bushel. You know how to take meaningful steps toward living the values closest to your heart, no matter what your inner critic might say. Your newfound self-confidence is a key that unlocks the cage where all your unique gifts have been trapped for so long. Now, you can show them to others—and every time you do, the world becomes a little better than it was before. The rest of us are so grateful that you chose to be seen.

RESOURCES

Acceptance and Commitment Therapy

The Happiness Trap by Russ Harris
Get Out of Your Mind and Into Your Life by Steven Hayes

Anxiety

The Anxiety Toolkit by Alice Boyes
How to Be Yourself by Ellen Hendriksen
Dying of Embarrassment by Barbara Markway, Cheryl Carmin, C. Alec Pollard, and Teresa Flynn
Painfully Shy by Barbara Markway and Gregory Markway
Anxiety and Depression Association of America: adaa.org

Body Image and Eating Disorders

Health at Every Size by Linda Bacon
The Self-Compassion Diet by Jean Fain
National Eating Disorders Association: nationaleatingdisorders.org

Cognitive Behavior Therapy

"50 Common Cognitive Distortions" by Alice Boyes. *Psychology Today*, January 17, 2013. www.psychologytoday.com/us/blog/in-practice /201301/50-common-cognitive-distortions
The Healthy Mind Toolkit by Alice Boyes
Cognitive Behavioral Therapy Made Simple by Seth Gillihan
Retrain Your Brain by Seth Gillihan

Confidence

Presence by Amy Cuddy
The Confidence Gap by Russ Harris
The Confidence Code by Katty Kay and Claire Shipman
The Confidence Code for Girls by Katty Kay and Claire Shipman

Depression

Beyond Blue by Therese Borchard
Uncovering Happiness by Elisha Goldstein
A list of resources to help with managing depression:
    www.everydayhealth.com/depression/guide/resources

Finding Help

"13 Qualities to Look For in an Effective Psychotherapist," by Susan Krauss
    Whitbourne. *Psychology Today*, August 8, 2011,
    www.psychologytoday.com/us/blog/fulfillment-any-age/20110
    8/13-qualities-look-in-effective-psychotherapist
Finding an ACT therapist:
    contextualscience.org/tips_for_seeking_therapist
Finding a CBT therapist: www.findcbt.org/xFAT
National Suicide Prevention Lifeline: suicidepreventionlifeline.org
    1-800-273-8255

Introversion

Quiet: The Power of Introverts in a World That Can't Stop Talking by Susan Cain
"The Power of Introverts." Susan Cain. TED Talk, February 2012.
    www.ted.com/talks/susan_cain_the_power_of_introverts

Mindfulness

True Refuge by Tara Brach
Advice Not Given by Mark Epstein
Meditation for Fidgety Skeptics by Dan Harris
The Road Home by Ethan Nichtern
Real Happiness by Sharon Salzberg
Review of meditation apps: www. healthline.com/health/mental-health
/top-meditation-iphone-android-apps

Resilience

Resilient by Rick Hanson and Forrest Hanson

Self-Compassion

Radical Acceptance by Tara Brach
The Mindful Path to Self-Compassion by Christopher K. Germer
Self-Compassion by Kristin Neff
The Mindful Self-Compassion Workbook by Kristin Neff and
Christopher Germer
More on self-compassion, including an assessment: self-compassion.org

Stress

The Upside of Stress by Kelly McGonigal
"How to Make Stress Your Friend." Kelly McGonigal. TED Talk, June 2013.
www.ted.com/talks/kelly_mcgonigal_how_to_make_stress_your_friend

REFERENCES

Altucher, James. *Choose Yourself*. Scotts Valley, CA: CreateSpace, 2013.

Beck, Aaron T. *Cognitive Therapy and the Emotional Disorders*. New York, NY: Meridian, 1979.

Bennion, Lowell L. *Religion and the Pursuit of Truth*. Salt Lake City, UT: Deseret Book Company, 1968.

Brown, Brené. *Daring Greatly*. New York, NY: Avery, 2012.

Cain, Susan. *Quiet: The Power of Introverts in a World That Can't Stop Talking*. New York, NY: Crown, 2012.

Card, Orson Scott. *Speaker for the Dead*. New York, NY: Tor Books, 1986.

Center for Growth. "Common Cognitive Distortions." https://www.therapyin philadelphia.com/tips/common-cognitive-distortions.

Creswell, J. David, William T. Welch, Shelley E. Taylor, David K. Sherman, Tara L. Gruenewald, and Traci Mann. "Affirmation of Personal Values Buffers Neuroendocrine and Psychological Stress Responses." *Psychological Science* 16, no. 11 (November 2005): 846–51.

Cuddy, Amy. *Presence: Bringing Your Boldest Self to Your Biggest Challenges*. New York, NY: Little, Brown, 2015.

Cuddy, Amy. "Your Body Language May Shape Who You Are." Filmed June 2012 at TEDGlobal. Video, 20:56. https://www.ted.com/talks/amy_cuddy_your _body_language_shapes_who_you_are.

Dalai Lama. Twitter post, January 17, 2011. https://twitter.com/dalailama/status /26941573090508800.

Dweck, Carol. *Mind-set: The New Psychology of Success*. New York, NY: Random House, 2006.

Ellis, Albert. *Overcoming Destructive Beliefs, Feelings and Behaviors: New Directions for Rational Emotive Behavior Therapy*. Amherst, NY: Prometheus Books, 2001.

Furtick, Steven. Twitter post, May 10, 2011. https://twitter.com/stevenfurtick/status/67981913746444288.

Hanh, Thich Nhat. *Fear: Essential Wisdom for Getting Through the Storm.* New York, NY: HarperOne, 2012.

Harris, Russ. *The Confidence Gap.* Boston, MA: Trumpeter, 2011.

Harris, Russ. "Embracing Your Demons: An Overview of Acceptance and Commitment Therapy." *Psychotherapy in Australia* 12, no. 4 (August 2006): 2–8.

Hendriksen, Ellen. *How to Be Yourself.* New York, NY: St. Martin's Press, 2018.

Ilardi, Stephen. *The Depression Cure.* Cambridge, MA: Da Capo Press, 2009.

Jeffers, Susan. *Embracing Uncertainty.* New York, NY: St. Martin's Griffin, 2003.

Johnson, Elizabeth. "Carrie Fisher Talks about Mental Illness and Career." *Sarasota Herald-Tribune,* April 20, 2013. http://health.heraldtribune.com/2013/04/20/14065.

Kabat-Zinn, Jon. *Full Catastrophe Living: Using the Wisdom of Your Body and Mind to Face Stress, Pain and Illness.* New York, NY: Delacorte Press, 1990.

Kaiser Permanente Medical Group. "Distorted Thinking." https://mydoctor.kaiserpermanente.org/ncal/Images/Done-Distorted%20Thinking_tcm75-461044_tcm75-461044.pdf.

Kaling, Mindy. *Why Not Me?* New York, NY: Crown Archetype, 2015.

Kay, Katty, and Claire Shipman. *The Confidence Code.* New York, NY: Harper Business, 2014.

King, Stephen. *On Writing: A Memoir of the Craft.* New York, NY: Scribner, 2000.

Kluger, Jeffrey. "The 2010 Time 100: Edna Foa." *Time,* April 29, 2010. http://content.time.com/time/specials/packages/article/0,28804,1984685_1984745_1985506,00.html.

Kowan, Joe. "How I Beat Stage Fright." Filmed January 2014 at TED@State Street Boston. Video, 8:03. https://www.ted.com/talks/joe_kowan_how_i_beat_stage_fright.

Lidsky, Isaac. *Eyes Wide Open Overcoming Obstacles and Recognizing Opportunities in a World That Can"t See Clearly.* New York, NY: Tarcher Perigree, 2017.

Linehan, Marsha M. *Skills Training Manual for Treating Borderline Personality Disorder.* New York, NY: The Guilford Press, 1993.

Markway, Barbara G., and Gregory P. Markway. *Painfully Shy.* New York, NY: St. Martin's Griffin, 2001.

McGonigal, Kelly. *The Upside of Stress*. New York: Penguin Random House, 2015.

Miller, Henry. *Big Sur and the Oranges of Hieronymus Bosch*. New York, NY: New Directions, 1957.

Rogers, Carl R. *On Becoming A Person: A Therapist's View of Psychotherapy*. New York, NY: Houghton Mifflin, 1961.

Salahub, Jill. "Self-Compassion Saturday: Kristin Noelle." *A Thousand Shades of Gray*. September 7, 2013. https://thousandshadesofgray.com/2013/09/07/self-compassion-saturday-kristin-noelle.

Salzberg, Sharon. *Real Happiness*. New York, NY: Workman Publishing Company, 2011.

Salzberg, Sharon. *Real Love*. New York, NY: Flatiron Books, 2017.

Segal, Zindel. "The Mindful Way through Depression." Filmed January 2015 at TEDxUTSC. Video, 18:05. http://www.tedxutsc.com/portfolio_page/the-mindful-way-through-depression.

Van Gogh, Vincent. "Letter from Vincent van Gogh to Theo van Gogh: Drenthe, 28 October 1883." http://www.webexhibits.org/vangogh/letter/13/336.htm.

Walsch, Neale Donald. Twitter post, July 23, 2016. https://twitter.com/realndwalsch/status/756942147119611904.

Walton, Alice G. "Where Does Self-Confidence Come From?" *Forbes*, June 10, 2011. https://www.forbes.com/sites/alicegwalton/2011/06/10/where-does-self-confidence-come-from.

Zabelina, Darya L., and Michael D. Robinson. "Don't Be So Hard on Yourself: Self-Compassion Facilitates Creative Originality among Self-Judgmental Individuals." *Creativity Research Journal* 22, no. 3 (2010): 288–93. https://doi.org/10.1080/10400419.2010.503538.

Ziglar, Zig. *Biscuits, Fleas, and Pump Handles*. Dallas, TX: Crescendo Publications, 1974.

INDEX

ACKNOWLEDGMENTS

We would like to thank Susan Randol, our editor, for her guidance and support on this project. We're also grateful for Greg Markway, who read our drafts and let us know when our writing got too cheesy. Jesse Markway, who has both blessings and talents, is the link between us that made this book possible. And even though Celia jokes that her inner critics are named Negative Nancy and Neil, the truth is that her parents, Nancy March and Neil Ampel, have always supported her dream of writing a book.

ABOUT THE AUTHORS

BARBARA MARKWAY, PhD, is a licensed psychologist with nearly 30 years of experience and is the author of four other books. Her first book, *Dying of Embarrassment: Help for Social Anxiety and Phobia*, was named one of the most scientifically valid self-help books in a study published in *Professional Psychology, Research and Practice*. She has appeared on *Good Morning America* and the *Today* show, and was featured in the PBS documentary *Afraid of People*. Her work has appeared in the *New York Times*, *Chicago Tribune*, *Washington Post*, *Prevention*, *Essence*, *American Health*, *Real Simple*, *Live Happy*, and *Business Insider*. She has been heard on radio shows across the country and she blogs for *Psychology Today*. She lives in St. Louis, Missouri, with her husband, Greg. Learn more about Dr. Markway on her website, BarbaraMarkway.com.

CELIA AMPEL is a writer whose work has appeared in the *Miami Herald*, *South Florida Business Journal*, *Daily Business Review*, and other publications. She lives in Miami, Florida.

CPSIA information can be obtained
at www.ICGtesting.com
Printed in the USA
LVHW02s1201260918
591424LV00002B/2/P

9 781641 521482